# HIGH PERFORMANCE LIFE

**www.highperformer.co.uk**



ISBN: 978-1-8384855-0-4

**Disclaimer**

Care has been taken to confirm the accuracy of the information presented and to describe generally accepted practices. However, the author is not responsible for errors or omissions or for any consequences from application of the information in this book and make no warranty, expressed or implied, with respect to the currency, completeness, or accuracy of the contents of the publication. Application of this information in a particular situation remains the responsibility of the individual. Any regimes described may not be considered absolute and universal recommendations. The author has exerted every effort to ensure that all information in this text is in accordance with the evidence at the time of publication.

The information contained in this book is provided for general purposes only. It is not intended as and should not be relied upon as medical advice. The publisher and author is not responsible for any specific health needs that may require medical supervision. If the reader has underlying health problems, or has any doubts about the advice contained in this book, he/she should contact a qualified medical or other appropriate professional.

How to Thrive and Achieve Fulfilling Goals through the Six Keys to Optimal Human Performance

# HIGH PERFORMANCE LIFE

CATHY SPEED

*In memory of my mum and dad;*
*Vitality, passion, and perseverance.*
*Forever in our hearts.*

# CONTENTS

**Foreword** 9

**Preface** 11

**About the Author** 13

PART 1 **SETTING THE SCENE**

1 **Predicting Performance:** We Are All Performers 17

2 **Notes of Caution:** Black Boxes, Gurus, and Cognitive Bias 25

3 **The Apprenticeship Journey:** Learning, Mastery, and Expertise 31

4 **What Kind of Learner Are You?** 53

5 **Success Does Not Equal Perfect** 57

## PART 2 **THE SIX KEYS**

**6 Passion for the Purpose** 63

**7 Perseverance** 69

**8 Conscientiousness** 77

**9 Self-Efficacy** 87

**10 Self-Awareness** 95

**11 Vitality** 107

**12 Chronobiology:** Timing Is Everything 125

**13 Fitness** 133

**14 Fitness in the High Performance Athlete** 159

**15 Nutrition for Us All** 165

**16 Nutrition for Exercise and Recovery:** Guidance for More Serious Athletes 195

**17 Sleep to Succeed: Sleep Well, Perform Better** 205

**18 Technologies in Human Performance:** Useful Servants but Dangerous Masters 223

**19 Looking to the Horizon** 229

**Appendix** 231

**Glossary** 232

**List of figures** 236

**List of Tables** 239

**Endnotes** 242

**Acknowledgements** 264

# Foreword

Sports is a great teacher. I have been blessed to have had the opportunity to represent my country in sports for 24 years and it has taught me many things. In sport, and in life, I have witnessed extraordinary achievements of individuals and teams, amazing successes, exhilarating moments, and inspirational efforts, but also disappointing outcomes and situations of under-performance that seemed to come from nowhere.

Hence being able to have a deeper understanding of what human performance means and how can one optimise one's own performances would go a long way in helping individuals do well in any walk of life – personal and professional. The principles that are outlined in this book resonate with my own experiences relating to the fundamental characteristics of human performance that explain many successes.

All of us have goals in life. Both in our personal lives as well as in our professional lives, we all aspire to get better. The keys to achieving goals in life do not start and finish with inborn talent alone. The keys are driven from within but must be nurtured through support and guidance. By understanding what influences performance, we all can be better equipped to achieve our goals. Professor Speed has captured these principles really well in this book.

I have known Professor Speed for many years now. During my playing days, I have reached out to her for medical advice related to my injuries on numerous occasions and her inputs have always been very helpful. I have also witnessed first-hand her overarching 'holistic' (whole person) philosophy, caring and supporting the individual to become their own expert and to grow through optimising the key principles described in this book. Her research and work in the wide field of human performance, and her focus on caring, supporting, advising, and protecting individuals and organisations from the 'noise' that can surround the pursuit of performance shines through.

This is not a book solely for the individual performer, though it will serve that person well. It is for all who wish to help others to thrive and to flourish in any walk of life. It is a book that should encourage principles of learning, mentorship and fulfilment. It is a book for us all.

**Sachin R Tendulkar**

# Preface

*'So what's good, what's true?'* This is the question one of my first mentors posed at the beginning of every meeting we had in my early career as a physician. Decades later I am still considering the experiences I have in day-to-day life with that question in mind. The world has changed dramatically in my professional lifetime that has now spanned over three decades. So many advances in medicine, science, technologies, global networks, and communications have been seen. And yet there are many other changes that have had profound negative impacts on the human race and this planet where we serve as custodians. Changes in lifestyles, cultures, tolerance of others, expectations, priorities, our climate, environments, our health and well-being, and yes, our perceptions of what's good and what's true – these are all the great challenges of the world in the twenty-first century.

I should perhaps have seen a warning of such changes that were to come in the series title of my first (very small) book, *Fast Facts...*, in the late 1990s. People were beginning to want only the superficial facts about a subject (in this case musculoskeletal injuries). Many across the globe were beginning to live life at breakneck speed, ever demanding of technologies, instant (often fake) information, travelling, working, earning, and rarely taking time to stop and reflect. Until, that is, the world came to a grinding halt. Early in 2020 the Covid global pandemic arrived, and it continues to hold us in its steely grip in the spring of 2021 as I write these words.

The concept of this book and some of its content have long sat in my mind, waiting for me to let go of other distractions to attend to the subject with the respect and attention it deserves. That moment arrived early in 2020, when it occurred to me that it was the ideal time to have a positive focus in the early hours of each morning as dawn appeared, before facing the daily challenges of life in the times of a deadly virus.

Throughout my career I have spent a lot of time in high performance environments, and I have learned much about the realities of what makes us perform, 'what's good, what's true', and what's not so good and untrue. I have long known that the key things that matter to performance and outcomes apply to most of us, regardless of whether we are 'elite', and I constantly try to communicate that to the spectrum of people from a wide range of backgrounds whom I take care of, advise, teach, and/or mentor. This book is part of that mission.

In the past year, when people have been forced to slow down, many have had time to reflect on their own goals, how they live life, what they want to achieve, and what truly fulfils them. That's really what human performance is: getting the most out of what we put our energies into. In its truest sense, it is holistic ('whole person') fulfilment, thriving, getting the most out of the lives we live, in the world that we live in, amidst the challenges we face. Those who learn to perform better can help others to do so too. And so, if this book helps in a very small way to assist the process to 'being all we can be', that would be a worthy achievement.

# About the Author

**Professor Cathy Speed**, BMedSci, BMBS, Dip Sports Med, MA, PhD, FRCP, FFSEM, SFHEA, is uniquely qualified to write this book. She is a Consultant in Rheumatology, Sport, and Exercise Medicine. She is Lead Physician at the Fortius Clinic, London, and is Clinical Director of the Centre for Human Performance, Cambridge. She is also Professor of Human Performance at Cardiff Metropolitan University, UK. Beyond her expertise in clinical medicine, she also has an academic background in exercise physiology. She acts as an independent consultant adviser in the health and human performance technology sector.

She has played senior roles in elite sport for over twenty years, including acting as Chief Medical Officer to a number of them. She was a Senior Physician at the English Institute of Sport (2002–2017). Roles have also included Physician at a number of Olympic and Commonwealth Games and Chief Medical Officer to Team GB Holding Camp for the Beijing Olympic Games. Her client base stretches far beyond sport and includes a wide spectrum of corporate workers and executives, and people of all ages and across all walks of life.

Professor Speed has a very active role in teaching, research, and education in the fields of clinical medicine and human performance, and is very widely published. She has been Senior Research Associate and Isaac Newton Teaching Fellow in the Department of Medicine, University of Cambridge. She is a Senior Fellow of the Higher Education Academy, UK.

Her clinical interests include human performance and the use of exercise and performance sciences in disease prevention and management. She also has interests in fatigue, bone health, soft tissue injuries, and arthritis. Her clinical practice blends her expertise in rheumatology, sports medicine, and human physiology. She applies a holistic philosophy in the management of all of her patients, young and old.

**www.cathyspeed.co.uk**

# PART 1

# SETTING THE SCENE

# 1

# Predicting Performance

## We Are All Performers

*When it is obvious goals cannot be reached, don't adjust the goals, adjust the action steps.*

**Confucius**

### Life's Natural Chaos

*You've been under a lot of stress recently. You know you need to make some changes, try to de-stress a bit.* So you set yourself a fresh goal that many do in this situation: you are going to get fitter, lose a little weight, eat and sleep a bit better, and hopefully get back on the tennis court soon. It's a Saturday morning and you are on your home treadmill, the one that everyone else in the family uses except you. You are power walking a pre-set hills programme. The treadmill gets a little faster, the incline goes up. Your phone rings. You can hear your teenage children shouting at each other in the garden. You can also hear your email inbox pinging. The doorbell rings. Damn it; you aren't going to get time to finish your power walk. You press the slow button on the console. Nothing happens. Then the treadmill gets faster, and steeper; you can't keep up. You try to step off and for some reason you can't; you're trapped... Faster and faster, steeper and steeper, you start to fall...

You wake up with a start. It was a dream, but most of that dream was close to reality: you frequently set out to achieve something but the chaos of life makes it so difficult. It would be fine if all you had to think about was that one goal – wouldn't life be simple! But it isn't. Life for most of us involves some 'natural chaos'. The treadmill of life can feel out of control, but you still want somehow to achieve the goals you set yourself and live life in a fulfilling way. It all seemed so straightforward when you downloaded a fitness programme, decided to cut back on some calories, and bought some new trainers. You've even bought a new smartwatch to help you monitor your health, although you are not really sure what it's telling you. Then all the other demands in life got in the way – issues at work, late night finishes, challenges at home, increasing pressures, and you start to get stressed, and tired. No time for those walking sessions, and bang goes the new diet.

That goal you set yourself could be anything – learning a new language, improving your presentation skills at work, enhancing your leadership skills, or just feeling better. Even with life's natural chaos, you still want to achieve those goals, to perform well, maybe even become an expert... It is true for us all: we are *all* Performers. We perform at work, at home, in our hobbies, in our interactions, in any of the goals we set, in all we do in life. Sometimes we perform well, sometimes we do not, and often we do not stop to consider why or to arm ourselves with the knowledge and tools to make the process easier and the outcomes more fulfilling.

## The Meaning of Human Performance

'Human performance' means different things to different people, and to many it means nothing at all. Many associate it with elite sport, or with workforce productivity and the corporate agenda, but beyond these contexts, the term has little resonance with most human beings in relation to their own lives, aspirations, and goals. And yet human performance in its true sense is central to all of our lives.

Performing simply means '*to begin and carry through to completion*'.[1] It can relate to a single task, working towards a specific goal, or an event. It can also relate to a much bigger picture – a journey such as a career, raising a family, or living life as a whole. The 'human' bit is just that – it is all about that human being, their life, their goals, their fulfilment, and the positive connections they form with others. The point is, performing is typically associated with achieving, accomplishments, and often with winning; and while these are undoubtedly meaningful across a number of domains, performing is more than that. Performing is about the whole person, attaining fulfilment. It relates to deriving more from what that individual human being does: thriving, feeling empowered, and enjoying life's journey more.

That's what this book is about. By focusing on the bigger picture of what performing means and having a true understanding of what key things influence it, the performer is far more likely to be successful. The process is not about personal reinvention, being perfect, always coming out on top, or 'greatness'. It is about enhancing peoples' understanding of what makes them tick, what makes them thrive, what ingredients are really important, and how to get more out of life for the energy they put in. That's Holistic (whole person) Performance, and it applies to us all.

These aspirations that most human beings have, to achieve goals and to make the most of what we do, are not unexpected, but the challenge is how to get there. So few feel they have the time to stop and think about how they do things. And when they do, how do they make sense of all the information about health, lifestyle, behaviours, and performance? There is so much confusing information about what predicts success in different domains – sport, health, business, home life. There are so many factors proposed to be *the* thing that makes or breaks your destiny: inborn talent, various personality types and traits, secret science, the influence of a fitness/leadership/other guru, having the latest technologies... To make any inroads we have to filter the noise, distil the cascade of information, and find the evidence for what works.

Human performance is very big business. Billions of dollars are invested by corporates into wellness programmes, workplace well-being facilities, and leadership and employee performance programmes. The global wellness market is considered to be worth $4.7 billion annually,[2] and the global corporate wellness market alone is expected to reach $100 billion by 2027.[3] Individuals spent $38.28 billion on performance-related products such as self-help books, fitness, diet, health, and lifestyle-related tools in 2019, and this figure is expected to grow at a compound annual growth rate of 5.1% from 2020 to 2027 (pre-Covid estimates).[4] Furthermore, the digital technology sector that has created a culture of the 'quantifiable self' continues to grow at breakneck speed; the global digital healthcare market alone is expected to reach $385.8 billion by 2025 from an estimated market size of $103.1 billion in 2019.[5]

Some of these programmes and products undoubtedly can help the individual who is trying to improve how they function in one or more elements of their life, but unfortunately, many do not. Profiling systems that tell us our personality type that, we are told, determines how we approach life; programmes that focus on finding our 'natural talents' that dictate how we perform; tools that focus on one specific aspect of performance and propose to make us great by changing that one thing using their 'unique approach'; products that measure everything about us but leave us feeling confused – all such tools make the whole concept of improving human performance much more challenging and energy wasting than it should be, and without the results to show for it.

My aim in writing this book is to lay out the basic truths about human performance, to dispel the myths, and to provide clear insights into what matters. If we examine the evidence, take away pseudoscience, and rely on the facts, there are just Six Key Characteristics that predict an individual's performance across most spheres of life, whether it is in work, life, or play. These Six Key Characteristics are *not* inborn; they are mostly acquired, and we can therefore all attain them with the right insights and support. Individuals who learn to display these characteristics are much more consistently successful in, and fulfilled by, how they perform. These characteristics are not secret, they are few in number, they interact with each other, and we don't need complex tools to put them into action.

One of these characteristics is **Vitality** (chapter 11), which is a huge part of how we perform. Vitality is not just our health and well-being, but it is underpinned by our positivity, our energy. It is *aliveness*. It is the product of our physical, physiological, mental, and emotional states; it is whole-person performance fitness for work, life, and play. There is emphatic evidence for the importance of vitality in driving fulfilling performances through a number of pathways.

Critical as vitality is to performance, I have placed it last in the discussion of the Six Keys in this book. Why? Because my three decades of working in human performance have taught me that those who do well, the people who find achieving goals so much easier than others do, are those who also possess five additional important attributes: Self-Efficacy, Self-Awareness, Conscientiousness, Perseverance, and Passion. Not only do they strongly influence vitality to ultimately drive the engine of performance, they also have a big effect on performance in their own right. In the world of human performance and well-being, so much influence is placed on elements of vitality – the right fitness, nutrition, and sleep programme – but even those who manage to navigate through the minefield of information and misinformation still frequently fail because they lack the other five keys or even an awareness those keys exist. All Six Keys interact, so improving in one area can have significant effects on others: *the whole is greater than the sum of its parts.*

We start our discussion of the Six Keys with **Passion** (chapter 6). I don't mean you are impassioned (yet) as the reader, but rather, we need to discuss what passion brings to the performance table. Well of course we should start with this, right? Having passion, or love, for the activity and it's goal is not absolutely essential, but performing really well is a whole lot harder – unlikely actually – without it. I am placing passion first also to emphasise the important role that positive psychology plays in every element of human performance. Passion differs from motivation, which is the trigger to actions we take to persevere with our goal when things get tough. Hey, presto! Perseverance is the second key we discuss.

**Perseverance** means persistence, continued effort, and determination even in the face of setbacks (chapter 7). It strongly overlaps with conscientiousness, self-effectiveness and self-belief. That's why we next cover conscientiousness. **Conscientiousness** (chapter 8) is the only personality trait that consistently arises as a predictor of performance in different scenarios. It means being careful and diligent. It is associated with being neat, planning ahead, adopting a systematic approach, and being thorough. It is the only key that is partly inborn. Many groan when they hear of conscientiousness in relation to performing, and this might be why attempts have been made to call it something else or combine it with other keys. We're not going there; it dilutes focus and effort.

Next, if you have never really delved into what self-efficacy can do for you, take note of the chapter that follows conscientiousness. **Self-Efficacy** (chapter 9) means our belief in our ability to perform well in specific areas of life and to apply the necessary behaviours to achieve specific goals.[6] It reflects our belief in our abilities to *walk the walk*. It doesn't mean doing everything ourselves; it typically also involves how we access the support we need to reach our objectives, while remaining conscious that we are solely responsible for ensuring we achieve it.

**Self-Awareness** (chapter 10) means seeing ourselves clearly; how we think, react, and behave. Increasing self-awareness often allows us to make leaps and bounds in working towards our goals. It takes time, focus, and effort and partly involves gaining help from others and from examining our strengths and our weaknesses. It can be an empowering process.

Then finally, we arrive at **Vitality**. Hopefully incorporating a lot of the messages into your approach will be so much easier, having read about the other five keys.

I am sure it's clear by now: these Six Keys, the evidence behind their importance in predicting individual performance in many spheres of life, and how to assess them are the focus of this book. Given the Six Keys are not inborn, the process of their development relies on an apprenticeship: learning and experiential journeys that can ultimately lead to the development of *mastery and expertise*. Hence, before getting to each of the Key Six in turn, this is where we start. We will travel through areas of physiology, health, neuroscience, psychology, and education to gain insights into how we learn new skills and behaviours, before considering how the Six Keys work to influence outcomes.

This is not a self-help book. It is a book that lays the foundations of human performance, the science, the facts. It is a book that should empower the individual reader through helping them to understand what human performance means, the areas that matter, and the science behind the principles for optimising their own performances. It is also a book to empower leaders, to assist them in selecting and driving human performance programmes that make a difference to the people around them. So whether you are reading this book for yourself, for your family, for your organisation, for others whom you lead, or all of these, it should provide clear insights into what is important in helping people to perform better, to possess vitality, and to thrive.

If you understand it, you can own it.

# 2

# Notes of Caution

## Black Boxes, Gurus, and Cognitive Bias

Given the size and scope of the human performance industry, the science and pseudoscience, and the potential for significant financial rewards for those who make and deliver products, it is not surprising that there are potential pitfalls for the consumer. So before we continue, some notes of caution.

### Beware Black Boxes

In science, computing, and engineering, a *black box* is a device, system, or object that can be viewed in terms of its inputs and outputs, without any knowledge of its internal workings. Its implementation is 'opaque' (black).[7] The term is highly relevant to the commercial side of human performance, where products – be they technologies that, in this era of the quantifiable self, measure everything about us, or be they personality, strengths, resilience scores, or any other form of analysis that is proposed to reflect our abilities and potential. Whether these products have something to offer or not, the issue is transparency: What is the evidence that they do what they claim to do? Unlike tools that are used in the healthcare industry, there is no regulation on human performance technologies. For example, a range of systems claim to measure our recovery, readiness, or general health status on any given day, but without providing the evidence to prove their worth. On a more basic level, even basic measures such as sleep, heart-rate-based metrics, and blood oxygen level are now widely available on devices, but many are grossly inaccurate. Here is another example: there are a range of performance programmes delivered by companies to individuals and workforces that use tools (e.g., questionnaires) that are not evidence based – or if the evidence is there, it is not published. So it might be fun to go through a programme and be told a variety of things about yourself and how to behave differently as a result, but how do you know this is all worthwhile? As with many products, we must differentiate the good from the less good and the distinctly bad, and that can be a real challenge. Currently it is up to the consumer to determine the quality and relevance of this range of human performance products.

If your doctor scribbles a prescription, tears it from the pad, and offers it to you, while saying 'Try this. I've no idea whether it works as there's no evidence, it might have adverse effects, who knows... Oh! and it may turn out to be quite expensive', would you take it? I hope not! If a financial adviser says to you, 'Invest in this! I've no idea if it's a safe investment, and I'm not really sure what it actually means, but trust it anyway', would you invest in it? Again, I hope not! Nevertheless we do these things all the time. We buy into programmes and products without asking as much as we should, such as: Where's the information that makes this a good idea? We invest not just financially, but more often with committing our focus and energy that is sapped along the way. Thankfully, there is another way. It's called the evidence-based approach. Any user, be they individuals examining a product for their own use or leaders and coaches examining systems for their workforce, will serve their goals well by scrutinising what they are buying into. We should not have to be rocket scientists to understand the products we are about to use.

The steps to take are:

- Ensure you understand what you are trying to achieve by using that product. Set very clear goals.
- Understand it – seek a clear explanation of the tool.
- Seek the science – Has the product been tested? By whom? Has the developer published or presented materials in peer-reviewed environments to support the validity of the product?
- What other options are there?
- Will this product serve your goal(s)? How are the effects going to be measured?

## Beware Gurus

'Guru' is a Sanskrit term for a teacher, guide, expert, or master of a specific field.[8] In ancient Indian times, the term extended beyond this, to more than someone who teaches a specific type of knowledge, and referred to someone who acts as a counsellor, a sort of parent of mind and soul who helps develop values and experiential knowledge as much as specific knowledge, an exemplar in life, an inspirational source who reveals the meaning of life.[9] In modern times, those who claim to be 'gurus' are rarely the best option for support.

## Choosing a Coach, Mentor, or Guiding Expert

At some point in the human performance journey, many will select one or more 'teachers' to assist them, be they a business that hires an expert to guide a corporate performance scheme, or an individual who is seeking a sport/fitness coach or any other form of mentor. Making the right choice is imperative, and choosing badly will be potentially damaging. So how do you choose?

1 **Experience** This means experience that is specific to the goals you are setting.

2 **Credibility** Examine their background further. Look at their CV. What's their track record? What have they done in the past that makes them potentially suitable?

**3 Reputation** Two approaches: one is to ask your peers, and if possible even other experts in the field. If they could choose any expert to guide them, who would they choose? Second, find others who have engaged that expert, and ask for feedback.

**4 Instinct** Meet that expert, get a feel for their compatibility with you and/or your organisation.

**5 Goals** Set targets, outcome measures, and a system of monitoring progress and ensuring two-way feedback.

The risk of having support can be dependency, where the individual can become a passive recipient of information without being empowered to become their own expert. Any performance programme should prioritise individual empowerment as a key objective. Such empowerment comes from laying the foundations that relate to key predictors of performance, giving the individual the tools they need to pursue a range of different goals.

*Spoon feeding in the long run teaches us nothing but the shape of the spoon.*

**E M Forster**

## Beware Cognitive Bias

Our brains are complex and very powerful organs, but the way we think can often have its limitations, and one of these is *cognitive bias*. This is where there is an error in how we process and interpret information and we base our judgments on that error. It is often a result of our brain's attempt to simplify information processing, and it often involves us making rule-of-thumb judgments that help us reach decisions with relative speed. We use biased recall of events, and/or we are biased in the information we select to form our views. It is not the same as being illogical – it is more related to making decisions based on a biased selection of facts, choosing what is convenient to believe. The issue of cognitive bias is relevant to how we function in all domains of life, and there are plenty of examples of that in the world we live in right now.

Cognitive bias results in taking mental shortcuts (heuristics) that can be dangerous and wasteful in relation to any theme, including human performance. For example, we pay attention to some things while ignoring other elements in front of us that could significantly change our judgement. Or we may make judgments about our health – for example, considering our own excessive weight is all due to our genetics but for everyone else it's because of their diets and inactivity. Or everyone *else* needs seven to nine hours of sleep to perform well, or eating late at night has negative consequences for everyone except you. We may demonstrate *anchoring bias* in relying too much on the first piece of information we learn about a subject, or *confirmation bias* in selecting information that confirms our preset beliefs, or *accessibility bias* in selecting the first bit of information that springs to mind. There are many more examples, but the point is that our cognitive bias, our heuristic tendencies, limit our progress with learning, skill development, and making use of information that is provided to us that would help us perform better. It also makes us biased in our selection of tools to help us in the performance journey, and this is why many products in the field are popular without being effective. We are all human, and many start with a bias that is driven by their optimism that there is a hidden single secret, tool, or system that will allow them to attain health and well-being, a finely tuned body, or fitness, or that will enable them to effortlessly excel at work or play the perfect game of golf.

The tricks to limit cognitive bias are, in theory, simple – even just being aware of it has been reported to reduce cognitive bias by 29%.[10] Further reflection on how we make judgments and decisions and challenging our potential biases are the steps to take to limit those biases. In real life that's challenging, but as you read this book, challenge yourself and how you process and utilise the basic truths about human performance that are described.

# 3

# The Apprenticeship Journey

## Learning, Mastery, and Expertise

*"If people knew how hard I had to work to gain my mastery, it would not seem so wonderful at all."*

**Michelangelo**

Michelangelo di Lodovico Buonarroti Simoni, known by most simply as Michelangelo, is viewed by many as the greatest artist of the Renaissance, and by some as the greatest artist of all time. He excelled not only in sculpture but also in painting and architecture, and he gave to the world some of its greatest works of art and beauty. He may have been known as 'Genius', 'Master', 'il Divino'... but it was he who highlighted the incredibly dedicated hard work behind his mastery.

**Mastery** means 'having a comprehensive knowledge or skill in a particular subject or activity'. The term is often used synonymously with 'expertise', but in fact, expertise is mastery that translates to concrete,

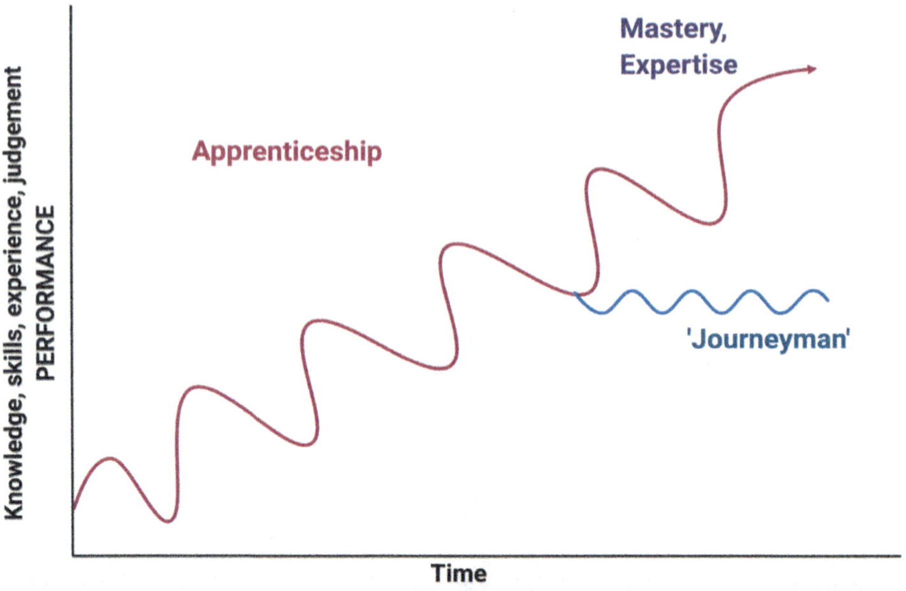


**Figure 3.1** The journey to mastery and expertise.

consistent, repeatable performances that are above and beyond what your peers achieve.[11] *It's walking the walk*. Arguably, only some masters become experts: those who not only have the acquired attributes of knowledge and skills in that field, but who are able to consistently produce top level results. But not all attain that mark: 'She knows a lot and has been in the business for years, but she just doesn't seem to be able to translate it to good outcomes'; or the pro golfer who has developed all the mastery components but when the stakes are high in a major tournament, they 'choke'. Hence, when the focus is on building mastery, having an awareness of the importance of translating that to performance is vital. The same factors drive both, but the focus on the key outcome of performance is the trick. What's the point otherwise?

The path to higher performance and ultimately to mastery and expertise is an apprenticeship. While many will not reach mastery levels, they still reach high levels of performance on the apprenticeship journey. In professional sport, those who stall in their development such that they reach a high standard but falter in reaching their highest goals are called 'journeymen'.

This book is *not* necessarily about becoming a master, nor an expert. It is about the processes that take us there, the apprenticeship, and the characteristics that determine the outcome of that journey, because anywhere along that route will mean enhanced performance. If the end result is mastery or expertise, then even better. Any path to enhancing performance in any domain is based on *how* we learn, *how* we develop knowledge and experience, reasoning, skills, and habits. So before we focus on the Six Key Characteristics, what we must first understand is how we learn to develop them.

## Experts Are Made, Not Born

Achieving mastery and becoming an expert is not about inborn talent. Having 'natural' skills – aptitudes that make people lean towards doing some things and away from doing others – will influence the paths chosen and the rate of learning and development. A person may lack hand-eye coordination but naturally lean towards creativity, and perhaps as a result be a better designer than an athlete. This doesn't mean that individuals cannot still improve their performance in sports and other physical challenges; and similarly those who don't feel they have much natural creativity can still gain much in that area if they have the desire to do so. Significant gains in any skill can be achieved through structured learning with the appropriate support, training, and practice. Furthermore, regardless of where the individual starts from in relation to natural aptitudes, everyone needs the opportunity to develop those skills, to get them started, even if that 'opportunity' is just an absence of barriers.

Broadly speaking, 'talent identification' programmes are usually disappointing. This does not stop their widespread use, especially in sport. These aim to identify those individuals who fulfil specific physical attributes that make them suitable to be streamlined into a particular sport at a young age, in the expectation they will become the sports stars of the future. Significant financial resources are invested in such programmes, but beyond recognising that height and weight might count in some sports, their effectiveness is questionable.[12] Furthermore, in other spheres of performance such as music, chess, and academic subjects, the evidence suggests that mastery is not so much about innate talent, IQ, or something else; it is all about learning, development, and mentorship that lead to the acquisition of knowledge, experience, reasoning/decision

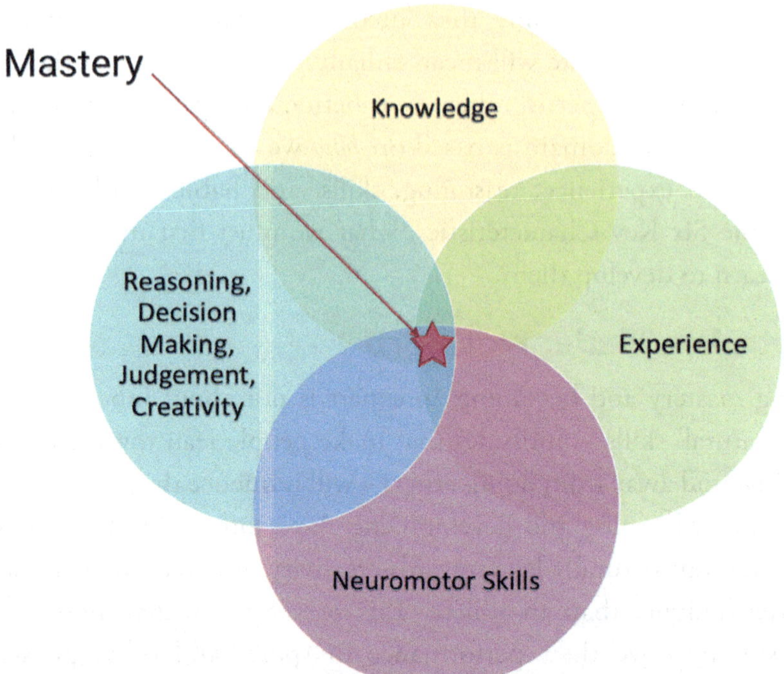


**Figure 3.2** Ingredients of mastery: Knowledge, motor skills, reasoning/judgement, experience.

making, and skills.[13] These are the ingredients of mastery and expertise, and their relative importance will differ across different disciplines in life. For example, the relative importance of motor skills is more significant in becoming good at a sport or becoming a surgeon, compared to those needed to be a great chess player or academic. Furthermore, those in creative professions such as architecture or design must train high-level mental skills that enhance creativity, which are facilitated in different parts of the brain than other cognitive functions, and result in a 'designer type' way of thinking and reasoning beyond just possessing knowledge. So we train the bits of the brain that are specific to the goals. We reap what we sow.

## The Journey to Performance: We Live, We Learn

The journey towards better performance, and to mastery, is dominated by the learning process that involves acquiring knowledge; gaining experience; and training various cognitive, reasoning, and motor skills. The main headquarters for this, of course, is our brain. 'Cognition', the processes that include thinking, knowing, remembering, judging, perception, planning, and problem solving, are all fundamental to performance and yet receive comparatively less attention in discussions about human performance. How we learn, how we gain the necessary knowledge and mental skills to perform, how other elements of our health and vitality like sleep, fitness, and nutrition affect our brains – these are all key to understanding how to perform in a sustained way in any domain.

## A Three-Minute Tour of the Brain in Relation to Performance

Our brains consist of different parts, called lobes, that are in general key centres for different functions. Take note of the frontal and parietal lobes. **Executive function** is largely based in the frontal lobe (especially the prefrontal area), while perception, spelling, and arithmetic are based in the parietal lobe (see figure 3.3). Executive function is a set of mental

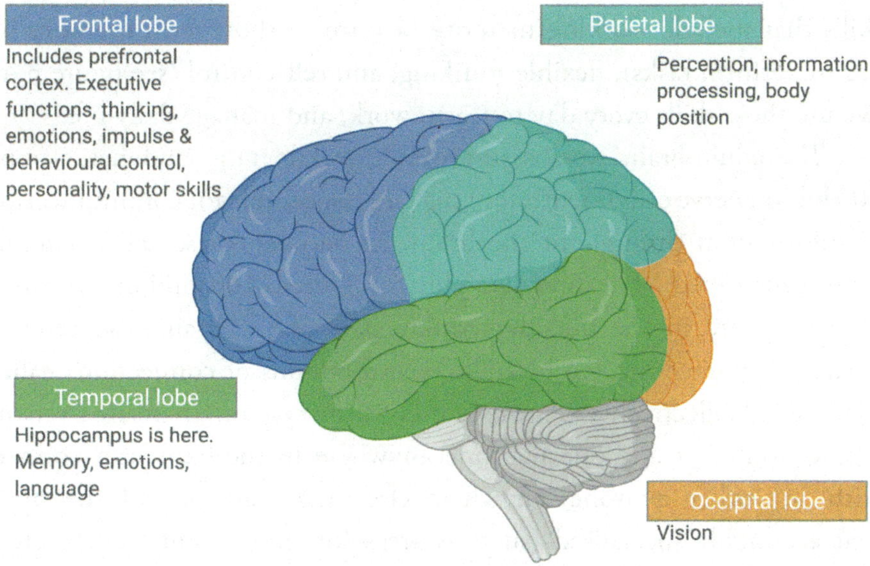


**Figure 3.3** The four lobes of the brain and their principal functions. (Executive function is based in the prefrontal cortex of the brain.)

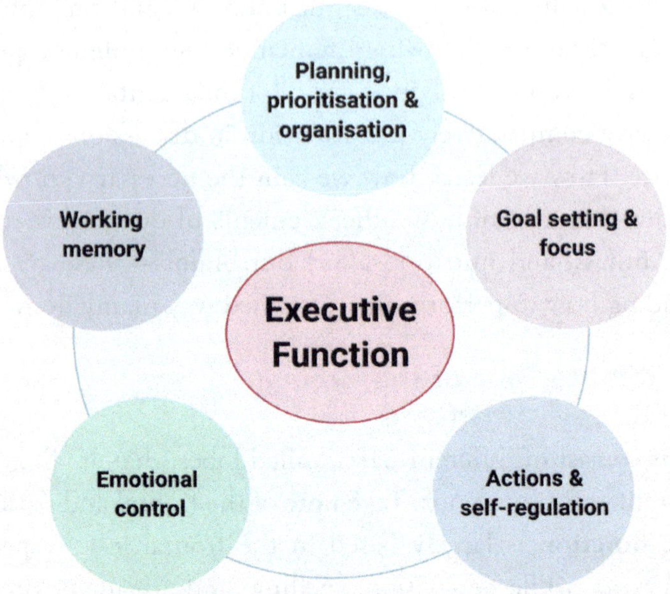


**Figure 3.4** The principal components of executive function, representing essential skills to perform in every domain of life.

skills that include working memory (a form of short-term memory we use to perform tasks), flexible thinking, and self-control (see figure 3.4). We use these skills every day to learn, work, and manage daily life.

The adult brain weighs just over one kilogram, and has around 100 billion nerve cells ('neurones') that are responsible for communication of information throughout the brain. In between these cells there are other cells called 'glia' (literally, 'glue'). Of these 100 billion neurones, 30 billion are in the outside wrinkly part of the brain, the cerebral cortex, all interconnected by billions and billions of connections called 'synapses'. Collectively that's the brain's wiring system. There are so many connections that any one neurone anywhere in the brain can connect with any other neurone, anywhere else. There are bits of the brain that are highly specialised (such as areas for smell, sight, touch, etc.), but most (>90%) of the cortex is developed to specifically ensure that, where needed, the cells can connect with each other. This is called the 'association cortex' and note this: the wiring system is not fixed; it adapts to all sorts of stimuli and also to use. Necessary linkages form through

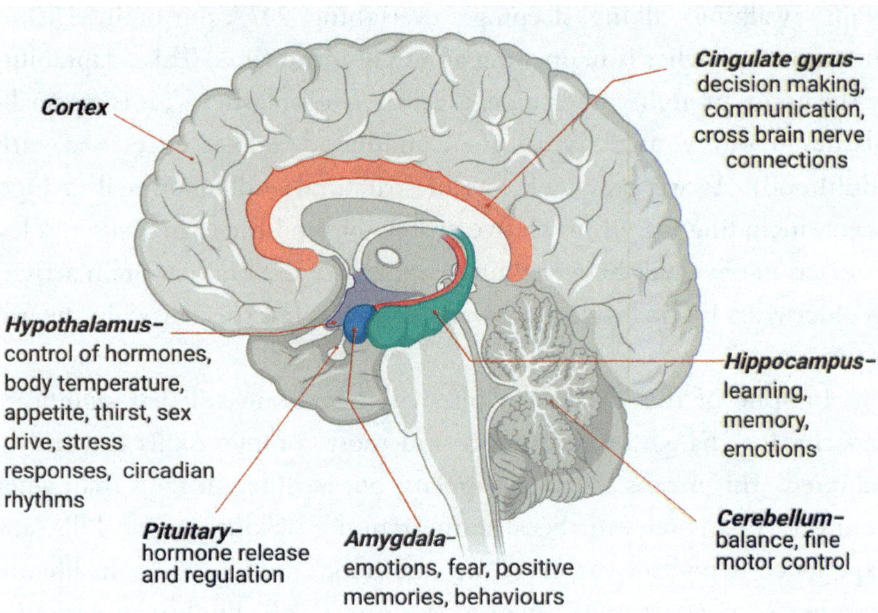


**Figure 3.5** A side view of important structures in the brain.

performing a task properly, time and time again, and this is partly how practice works; it develops the necessary circuitry to perform. Circuits develop not only across areas of the cortex, but also between the cortex and other areas of the brain, including the cerebellum, which controls movement and balance. So if we take up a new hobby, let's say ballroom dancing, there is a lot to process – where our body is in space, where our feet are, hearing the music, identifying the rhythm, planning, movement, synchronising with our partner – and all of this starts with messaging connections between various parts of the brain. The more we practice, the more we stop thinking about what we are doing; we are reaching *automaticity*, which in some areas of performance is essential. Notably, when we consider executive function based in the prefrontal cortex, this area has numerous connections across *several* areas of the brain, including the cerebellum, where balance and fine motor control are partly based.

These changes can occur because the brain is 'plastic'; it is constantly changing in response to how we use it, our environment, experiences, our genetics, and where in our life cycle we are. Everything we do changes our brain – walking, talking, sleeping... everything, 24/7; our brain cells fire in response to what is happening at any point in time. This adaptability of the brain, its ability to change, is called 'neuroplasticity'; it is especially plastic in our younger years (i.e., childhood, adolescence, and early adulthood). As we get older, lots of structural and functional changes occur, including loss of protective protein around the brain cells and less interaction of signals between different parts of the brain.[14] Brain activity in older years is also less localised, meaning it is less specialised in the way it functions.[15]

In spite of this decline in plasticity, the brain still has significant capacity for change in adulthood, and most complex skills can still be acquired. This means learning happens, but at different rates than when younger. This is relevant because the refining of knowledge, skills, and experience is typically achieved in adulthood, and engaging in lifelong learning is a necessity, not a luxury. This process of adult learning is called 'andragogy' (literally, 'leading adults'). As adults, we may learn more slowly than when younger, but learning is greatly assisted by experiences we have had along the way, and so we learn more by using reasoning and problem-solving approaches than memorising facts. As we get older, we also have a greater independence in our learning and have different motivations and more focused objectives. It follows that when learning in groups, interaction between those at different stages in their lives can bring fresh perspectives.

Neuroscientists have provided much insight into *how* we learn, how the brain responds and adapts. They use Magnetic Resonance Imaging (MRI) to measure the volume of areas of the brain, functional MRI (fMRI) to demonstrate brain activity by detecting changes in blood flow, and Positron Emission Tomography (PET) to measure metabolic activity in the brain. Electroencephalography (EEG) can directly demonstrate electrical activity in the brain (essentially 'brainwaves' generated by the brain cells) through electrodes placed at multiple sites on the scalp. Hence, there are ways of looking at how the brain changes with learning across different domains – simple and complex motor skills, languages, maths, music, and so on.

Research using fMRI has shown that the brain activity of children is significantly different in those who are musically train compared to those who are not.[16] Furthermore, research also shows that music training enhances executive function skills.[17]

Just as a muscle adapts to training, so does the brain, and studies with MRI have given some insight into what actually happens when this occurs. There is a well-known study of London taxi drivers who have to pass 'the Knowledge' – exams that relate to the intricate layout of London and how to navigate around its 25,000 streets.[18] They sit a number of tough exams to get their license, with a pass rate of around 50%. Firstly, the research team demonstrated that these drivers have greater brain volume in the hippocampus, the region of the brain that controls memory and navigation skills. They then monitored 79 drivers from the beginning of their learning over a four-year period, and another 31 people who did not drive taxis but were of similar age, education, and intelligence as the taxi trainees were also studied. At the start of the study, all of the participants had more or less the same size hippocampi and performed similarly on tests of working memory and long-term memory. Of 79 drivers, 39 passed the Knowledge tests and gained their licenses. Of those who failed, 20 agreed to continue to be studied. Drivers who earned their licenses performed far better in memory tests than those who failed – even though they had performed equally four years earlier. Furthermore, MRIs showed that the successful trainees' hippocampi had grown over time. That increase in size might be due to more brain cells forming, or more connections developing between them, or both. Either way this is a big deal; cognitive training can cause physical and wiring changes in the brain. Further research has shown that, in those individuals with exceptional memories, there is *no association with IQ*. They simply train memory skills over time, such that fMRI scans have shown increase in the activity of the hippocampus in these people.[19]

To further explore the way the brain adapts to facilitate better performance, let's take a specific domain of learning, arithmetic, which is an essential component of functioning in life. We don't process numbers in a uniform way; the way our brains deal with numbers actually depends on the type of problem in front of us, and which bit of our brain we use depends on the complexity of the tasks and the training we have been exposed to. Simple calculations are performed in the left parietal lobe of the brain, and more complex calculations seem to involve parts of the frontal lobe and other areas too. We have specific wiring, circuits within these areas, that deal with specific problems presented to us. When we undergo short-term intensive training in arithmetic problems, we get faster and more accurate, and this is related to significant changes in brain activation patterns. As we learn, there is a shift from slow and effortful processing within the brain to skilled and fast retrieval, and the more expert we are, the more things we simply store in our memories, which is located in different parts of our brain to that used for actually effortfully processing a calculation. So as an expert, you don't need to drain energy in processing a calculation to get the answer; it's kept in easy-access storage. Training helps you to conserve energy, and energy conservation as a whole is important in maintain any high performing state. Other studies have reinforced this. One study assessed young adults given five days of intensive training on complex mathematical problems.[20] Findings indicated rapid improvements in response times and accuracy. The longer the training, the faster and more accurate the participants' performance. With practice, complex arithmetic becomes not only faster and more accurate, but involves less brain activity in the prefrontal region (the complex calculation site) of the brain to achieve it. More evidence that it gets easier and less energy-consuming.

Moving beyond a purely thinking task, what about the process of learning and performing more motor-orientated skills, such as in sport? Consider hitting a tennis ball. The process involves seeing the ball; positioning yourself in space; swinging the racket; making a judgement as to where you want to place it, deciding what sort of shot you want to make, how much spin, where to position yourself after you've hit the shot; judging where your opponent will be, etc. This requires training not only of motor skills, but also perception and decision making – all processed in split microseconds across multiple interconnected parts of the brain. In studies of elite athletes, it is clear that training in the form of deliberate practice (discussed further below), results in significant changes in the structure and wiring of these areas.[21] Not only are motor skills trained, but there is an enhanced ability through this training to predict how events will unfold, based on the movements of our opponents, and to use these predictions to increase the speed and accuracy of our decisions and of our actions.

Take another example, a more extreme one: the brain of fighter pilots, who have to process multiple sources of information and make precision decisions while flying the plane at speeds up to 1,500 mph while operating under high G-forces, still staying aware of the changing environment around them. It is a discipline that is considered to be at the limit of human cognitive capability since it requires skills of fine control with minimal space for error.[22] Research shows that the brains of fighter pilots are wired very differently.[23] Their brains show greater accuracy and enhanced processing of information for goal-driven decision making. They are also more sensitive to distracting stimuli, which probably reflects the need to be 'hyperaware' in their environments. MRI scans show the structure of their brains differ from the control, with relevant areas of the right side of the brain being larger and connections between key areas in the brain laid out differently. Nature or nurture? Given the evidence of the effects of training on the brain, it's probably more the latter.

And a final example, the brains of those with skills relating to high creativity versus those without. The neural network, the wiring, of the high creativity group's brains show much greater dense networks especially in the fronto-parietal region, including in the area where executive function is largely based.[24] How that specifically results in high creativity is not clear, but the point again is that the wiring develops according to the purpose.

## Staying Brain-Fit

Just like physical attributes that come with fitness training, maintaining cognitive fitness – essential to performance – is a case of use it or lose it. For example, when the London taxi drivers mentioned earlier retire, their increased brain volume shrinks. Similar changes have been seen in the acquisition of other skills such as juggling, playing music, and dance. In one research study, when a group of young adults were taught a three-ball juggling routine for three months and then scanned after they had become skilled performers, certain parts of their brains had changed in response to the training, and there was a close relationship between the extent of the change and performance.[25] When the jugglers were then 'detrained' for three months (meaning they did not perform any juggling in this time) and then were scanned again, their brain changes had disappeared, and the increase in brain volume that had been seen had declined.

Another study relating to brain plasticity assessed an older group of adults (mean age sixty years) who were taught to juggle.[26] With training, very similar changes in brain structure in comparison to younger adults were seen, but they acquired less skill for the same change in brain volume; so possibly as we get older, we need to acquire more structural change in our brains to achieve the same outcome. It is not just motor skills that are different as we age; learning a new language, for example, is slower than when we are younger. Adults differ considerably in these changes in neuroplasticity and rates of learning, partly for genetic reasons, partly due to their environment, and partly due to their health. As will be discussed later, exercise, sleep, and nutrition all have major impacts on how the brain works and adapts. It is another reason why vitality is central to performance. Similar to other aspects of health and fitness, the brain also needs training, regular 'brain exercise', to keep adapting to challenges.

Even just thinking, seeing, or hearing certain familiar stimuli can increase activity in certain parts of the brain that are charged with performing a particular task. So in a tennis player, parts of the brain that control specific muscle contractions representative of movement on court are activated in response to the player being shown videos of playing tennis, and this has relevance to practice using visualisation techniques to improve skills.

## Deliberate Practice and the '10,000 Hour Rule'

Central to the development of mastery and becoming an expert is deliberate practice – goal specific, purposeful, planned, focused, systematic practice that is supervised and/or supported by mentorship of some form. The resulting rate of development of expertise varies across individuals and across different tasks. In 1899 the authors of a study of Morse code telegraphists proposed that it takes ten years to become an

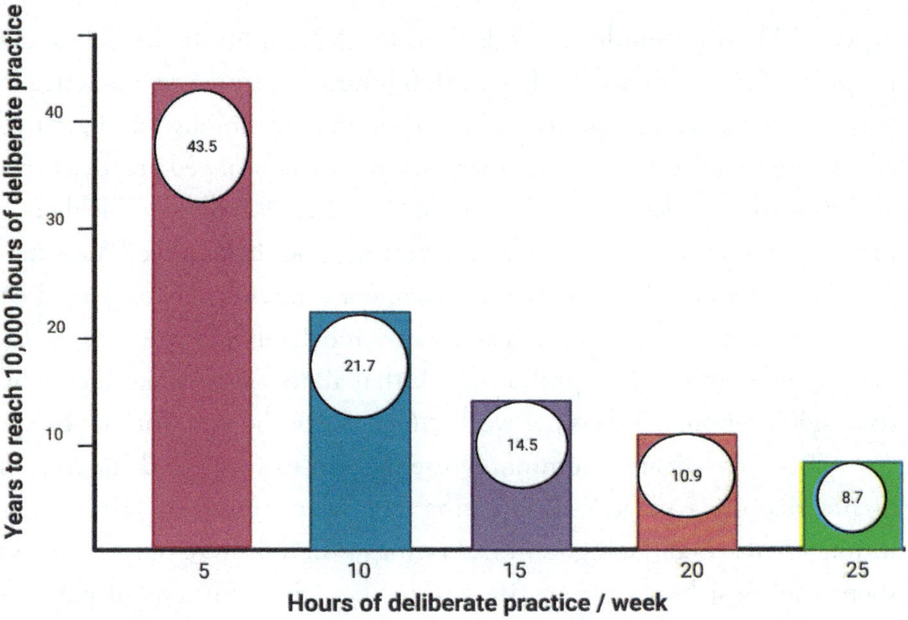


**Figure 3.6** Number of years to reach 10,000 hours of deliberate practice, based on practicing 46 weeks/year.

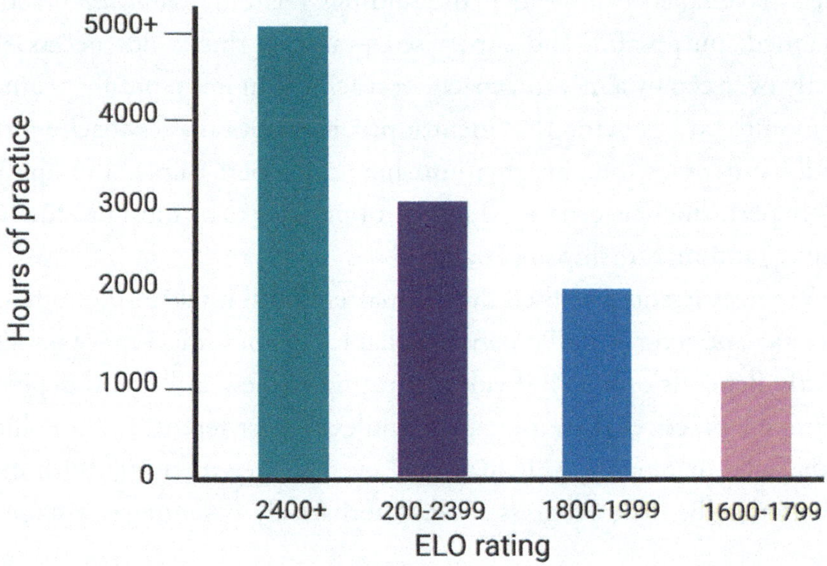


**Figure 3.7** The most successful chess players have put in significantly more hours of practice.[27]

expert.[28] Almost a hundred years later in 1993, Ericsson and his colleagues proposed that in essence it takes 10,000 hours of training and practice to become an expert in a specific field.[29] They studied violinists and pianists and found that musical prowess increased with accumulated practice time. Top-ranked violinists had on average achieved 10,000 hours of deliberate practice by the age of twenty. Researchers in other fields have found that 10,000 hours of deliberate practice have commonly been completed by those who achieve expertise across a range of disciplines, including sport, music, chess, and various professions. Is that all that surprising? It equates to roughly 5 hours, 5 days per week, 46 weeks of the year, for 10 years.

Chess players are a commonly used group to study, and the impact of practice on a player's ELO rating[i] has been examined. Those who ultimately reached the highest ELO ratings (>2,400) were those who had spent the most hours of practice within their first ten years of playing, versus significantly less time spent by those at lower skill ratings.

Unfortunately, the '10,000 hours rule' has been highly popularised and oversimplified in the process and has sparked *much* debate and misunderstanding. Some have assumed this is a strict rule, rather than a well-researched rule of thumb with some common sense behind it. Others have failed to note that the findings relate to *deliberate* practice – planned, purposeful, and supervised practice. This is not necessarily directly overseen by a mentor, coach, or teacher, but it is typically planned and monitored by them. That mentor provides not only feedback on the practice outcomes, but insights into how an expert thinks and applies skills in performance scenarios. Hence, for practice to be most productive, coaching and mentorship are key.

When Ericsson proposed that to master a skill it takes 10,000 hours of practice, he actually said it *may* take that long. For some it may take less. It partly depends on our individual learning curves, and it also depends on *how* we practice. If we practice mindlessly, just repeating something for the sake of repetition, it may take even longer than 10,000 hours, or there may be little progress at all. Alternatively if we practice *smart* –

i. The Elo rating system is a method for calculating the relative skill levels of players in zero-sum games such as chess. It is named after its creator Arpad Elo, a Hungarian-American physics professor.

purposefully and deliberately – then we will be more efficient and achieve more satisfying outcomes. Investigate the stories of any expert, and you will hear similar experiences relating to focused practice. Whether it's the micro-skills involved in becoming a sushi chef, the path to becoming a surgeon, the journey to becoming a chess Grandmaster, the process is the same: practice deliberately or you won't make it.

It is fair to argue that deliberate practice is not *all* that counts. If we compare a group of Formula 1 racing drivers or tennis pros, we find most have done their 10,000 hours of deliberate practice, and often much more – but some become are more successful than others. Then there is perhaps the true occasional outlier. In chess, Gobet and Ereku highlighted the case of Magnus Carlsen, a highly atypical chess Grandmaster, who was not only No. 1 in the world in 2014, but he was truly miles ahead of the rest, with the points gap between him and the No. 2 player being the same as the differential between the No. 2 and No. 14 players at the time.[30] Carlsen's rating was 100 points ahead of the No. 10 player in the world, statistically representing half a standard deviation in skill, giving him a probability of winning of 63.7%. By this time he had been playing eighteen years (though he started to play seriously at the 'old' age of eight, so that's thirteen years of serious focus). Carlsen's training behaviours are *not* known, but it is said he only practices in a way he enjoys, and it is not structured, and so it is not 'deliberate'. There will always be the occasional exception to every rule.

On the basis of the 10,000 hour proposal, we might expect that expertise should increase with age, as the latter should reflect the amount of experience gained. That is true for some areas; for example, research has shown that the skills of surgeons completing a specific operation improve with age.[31] However it is not true for some others professions, such as physicians, whose expertise increases initially then can start to decline with increasing age.[32] It may be that age in some professions is not a good surrogate marker for experience – implied by the fact that physicians' performances are better in those who have busier practices, even though age since graduation was correlated with poorer outcomes.[33] Furthermore, the inconsistent effects of age may relate to some professionals dedicating less time to knowledge building and staying up to date as they take on more leadership and/or administrative responsibilities within their field. It is also influenced by how our brains work and the changes in learning capacities as we age. If nothing else, this highlights the need for experts and leaders to continue to follow the discipline that got them there in the first place, to dedicate time to learning, and to get the mentorship and support they need, no matter how senior they are. That's why it's called *continuous* professional development.

The evidence clearly suggests that deliberate practice strongly impacts the process of developing the key elements of mastery and becoming an expert. What are the key factors that drive the ability to commit to the process, to reap the benefits, and to continue through the challenges of apprenticeship? They are the Six Key Characteristics that predict successful performance (see figure 3.8).

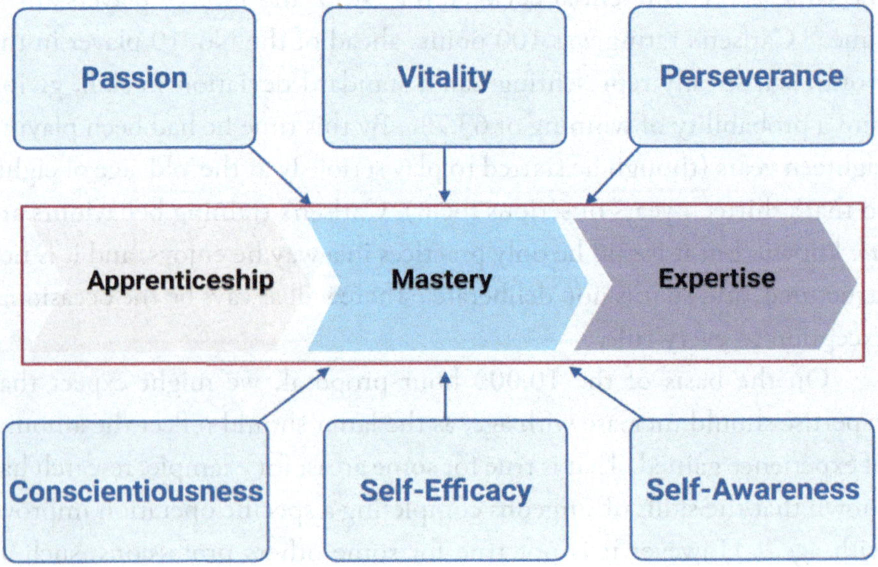


**Figure 3.8** Six Key Characteristics of Performance drive the development of mastery and expertise.

## Real world expertise:
## **The great fire of Notre Dame, 2019**

On 15 April 2019, just before 18:20 on a beautiful spring day in Paris, an electrical short circuit created a spark high up in the largely wooden attic roof ('the forest') of Notre Dame Cathedral. The fire alarm rang shortly afterwards and the cathedral was evacuated. But when a security guard went to investigate, he inspected the wrong area, and he found no fire. He was new on the job and was on his second eight-hour shift that day because a replacement colleague had not arrived for his shift. Initially some visitors were allowed back into the building. Fifteen minutes passed before some guards became concerned and climbed the 300 steps up to the roof space to look further. There they could see the fire had taken hold and summoned the fire brigade, who arrived ten minutes later. Ultimately, 400 firefighters were involved in fighting the fire, ranging from junior staff to seasoned professionals, team leaders, and commanders. All possessed the necessary knowledge base of firefighting, had passed essential training, and had vital skill sets to perform their job well. Each were at a different place on their performance journeys – some were highly experienced, and others had many years of focused training under their belts. All played their roles that day.

Leading the 400 firefighters was General Jean-Claude Gallet. At fifty-four years of age, he was an expert in his field; he had served in Afghanistan and specialised in crisis management. A knowledgeable and highly experienced expert, he had to make reasoned, rapid decisions in an ever-changing situation. He strategized with his team on how best to tackle the flames, knowing he could not use aerial water as it would damage the cathedral structure further, and he could not get images from helicopters due to the threat of the flames. He armed himself with information provided by his team, by other experts, and by drones, robots, and thermal imaging.

Teams of fighters worked initially from within the building, exhibiting key features of high performance: conscientiousness in following technical protocols, self-awareness and self-efficacy in their actions to push back the fire, and making judgement decisions on how to safely position themselves best to push back the flames, having the positivity and physical strength and endurance to continue with their mission, and above all persevering. But the fire continued to win the battle. At 19:50, with the fire spreading, the iconic wooden spire of the cathedral collapsed. Shortly before this, the fire spread to the northern tower of the cathedral, where wooden framework supported eight huge historic bells.

Gallet recognised the significance of the fire in the north tower: if the roof burned, the bells (supported by wooden structures) would fall, and likely take the rest of the cathedral with it. Experience told him that he had less than twenty minutes before this would occur, and that unless he adopted a different strategy, the results would be catastrophic. He and his team devised a new and highly daring approach, involving a team of firefighters scaling the towers at the front of the building, then attacking the fire from within the towers. Gallet drew on his knowledge, judgement, reasoning skills, flexibility, and experience to make strong decisions and to guide his team, and his team drew from their own learning and experiences to carry out the challenging work involved.

Success! At 21:45 the fire came under control; the towers and the cathedral were saved. Many hours of fighting the fire followed before the firefighters finally returned to their stations in the early hours of the morning. Some had a station inspection at 06:00 the next day, and in spite of having just battled the biggest fire of their lives, they conscientiously worked on for a few hours, cleaning equipment to be prepared for their next challenge.

So what's the point of this story? Firstly, maybe the fire took greater hold partly because the initial inspection was carried out by a fatigued, and possibly inexperienced, sole security guard, faced with making a difficult decision of whether to persevere with his search. Secondly, only an expert like Gallet could have made those experienced judgements that saved the cathedral; judgement that had evolved over years of training and experience. Thirdly, only a team of highly trained firefighters, all on their apprenticeship journeys, some masters, but nevertheless all high performers in their respective roles in an immensely stressful situation, could have got the job done. On the apprenticeship journey to mastery and expertise, we can all be very highly effective Performers.

## Learning Curves and Great Expectations

When we enter a learning/training programme, an apprenticeship, we have expectations or strong beliefs that something is going to happen. In the context of performance, this is typically associated with achieving a goal within a certain timeframe and through a specific process. Anyone who is involved in such a programme has expectations, whether it is for themselves or for their team: expectations of the individual, expectations of others, of the size and speed of changes that are involved, and of the outcomes.

Within all of the debate about needing 10,000 hours of deliberate practice, little discussion seems to relate to what the journey often looks like. Frequently it is peppered with unexpected setbacks. This is a necessary and inherent part of the learning process: '*Success does not consist in never making mistakes but in never making the same one a second time*'

*No one is so brave that he is not disturbed*
*by something unexpected.*

**Julius Caesar**

(George Bernard Shaw). This is why, as will be discussed, self-effectiveness, perseverance, and positivity are crucial: they help to manage those setbacks and maintain the momentum to progress in the right direction. Having mentorship and a good and motivated support team helps to support that process.

Managing expectations, monitoring progress, and keeping an eye on performance is facilitated by using learning curves, and adapting them where needed along the way. Learning in various ways is inevitably central to developing mastery, and as has been mentioned, the rate of learning can vary across tasks and people, so in the context of human performance these curves can be personalised and adapted as the individual progresses.

The concept of learning curves, if not the term, was initially proposed by German psychologist Hermann Ebbinghaus in 1885. His interest was in the study of memory; he tested memory of nonsense syllables and recorded the success across repeated trials, showing it in the form of a learning curve.[34] Subsequently, learning curves were developed for the evaluation of learning of individuals in many settings as well as being used in predicting manufacturing production turnover, machine learning, and economic modelling.

Learning curves may be short or long and simple or complex. So if you look at figure 3.9, you see that curve A (short) relates to a skill that is easy to acquire, and the rate of learning is rapid (steep). Hence, although the term 'steep learning curve' is often used to describe a difficult learning process, it really means a learning experience that involves a *rapid* gain in the skill, as in curve A or part of curve C. Curve B shows a slower rate but potentially more to gain at the end. Curve C is a sigmoid 'S' curve, which shows a slow start, then a rapid rise, and then a slowing of further skill acquisition. It may be those last few increments that make someone a true expert. Learning curve D is a complex curve, showing a slow start, plateau, then a rapid increase. The message is that learning curves can come in all shapes and sizes and can change as the process moves forward.

There is the potential at the late stage of any of these curves for *automation*, where the skill becomes a habit, demanding little if any conscious thought to do it. For many elements, particularly motor skills, that's a good thing. For other skills that depend on thinking, reasoning,

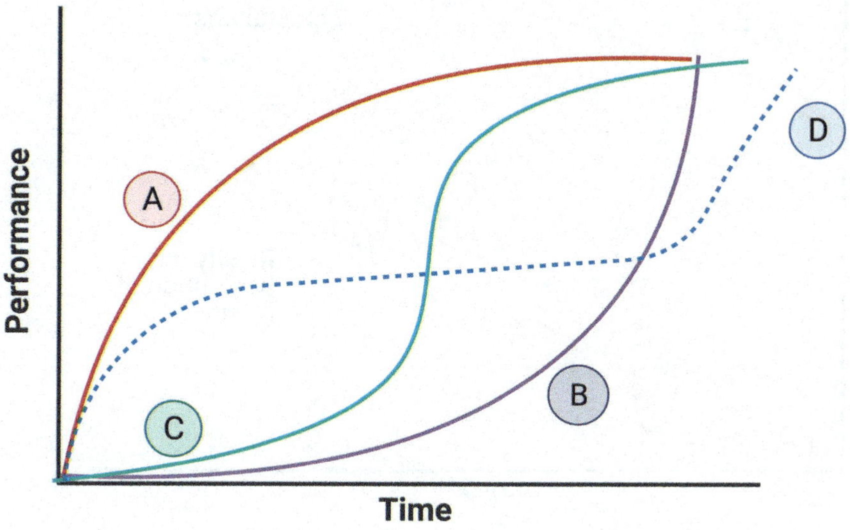


**Figure 3.9** Learning curves vary significantly across individuals and tasks.

and judgment, doing things on autopilot is dangerous. So, although we don't want a fighter pilot to be thinking too long about the process when he sees an unexpected hazard in front of him, I for one don't want the last few words I hear from my surgeon before I go under an anaesthetic to be, 'Don't worry, I am on autopilot...'

The key message is that learning curves should be used from the outset, discussed along the way, and adapted when needed. They can enhance motivation and allow a focus for discussion with mentors in relation to progress towards a goal. Otherwise we end up with the curve E in figure 3.10 (*overleaf*), which is how it might feel to the learner if expectations are not managed.

## Making Sense of It All

What are the key messages we can take from all of this? Firstly, embracing and engaging with lifelong learning is a fundamental criterion to performing well, and figuring out how to do this effectively is the key. How our brains respond to stimuli determines how we learn and how we perform; those responses are individual and change through life. The brain is exercised by, and responds to, deliberate practice, and the role

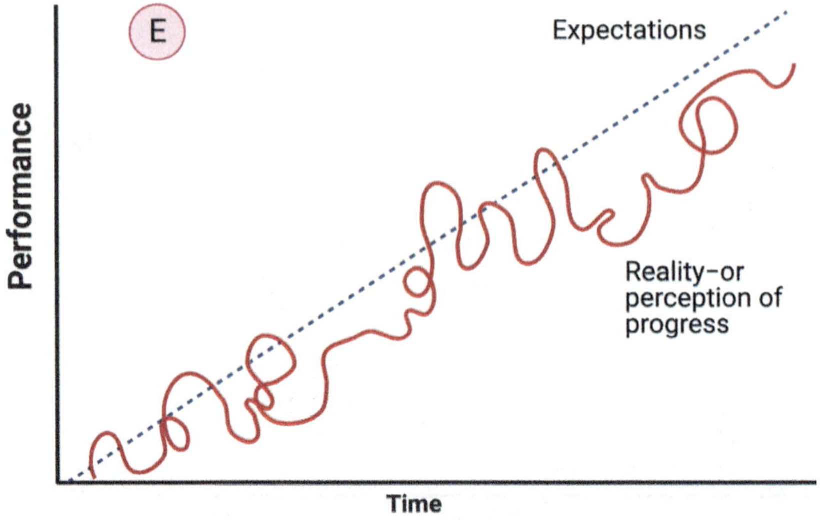


**Figure 3.10** How the learning process may feel to the learner if planning is inadequate and/or expectations are not managed.

of any coach or mentor is to help tease out what the individual will best respond to. How we learn, our brain plasticity, is also influenced by our own actions; exercise, sleep and nutrition all play a major role, and they will be discussed further in chapter 11, 'Vitality'.

Secondly, brain training must be ongoing. Use it or lose it.

Thirdly, the more we practice, the easier it gets – literally. We draw on memories from practice rather than having to use the energy to process thoughts.

Fourthly, the best learning and performance programmes for individuals and groups allow for the fact that there are differences in how our brains are wired, and that our age and our physiology contribute to learning curves that are different across individuals. Having a learning curve in mind, and monitoring it, is a smart part of getting the most out of training.

# 4

# What Kind of Learner Are You?

*Tell me and I forget, teach me and I may remember, involve me and I learn.*

**Benjamin Franklin**

*Lifelong learning* may sound intimidating, but we are all learning throughout our lives. Every day we assimilate masses of information, we process it, learn from it, act on it. It takes quite a lot of our energy, and so it is worth considering how we learn and how to make the process most effective and efficient.

We may all be constantly learning, but the way that we learn differs between us. Our learning styles really dictate whether we take on the information being given to us. A simple example: when those bookshelves that looked so great online arrive packed flat in a box, how do you figure out how to put them together? Do you read through the written instructions? Do you search for diagrams? Do you ask someone to show you or look for a YouTube video online? Or do you ask someone to talk you through it?

The subject of learning styles is controversial amongst educationalists, not because their existence is disputed, but rather because there are a whole range of different tools used to assess them. The best tool is one that not only defines the styles but also gives insight into how to use that information. The challenge is that if you are learning in a group, such as in a formal training setting or more likely in meetings, you can't expect others to provide information in a range of ways to accommodate the diversity of learning styles in the room. It is better that individuals are empowered through knowledge of their own learning styles to adjust to different situations.[35] This is *metacognition*, thinking about how you think, and it is part of self-awareness and will be discussed in chapter 10.

The **VARK** model of learning is a popular tool to establish an individual's learning styles.[ii] A reading/writing style is the most common, perhaps partly because this is a common teaching emphasis in schools. Many are multimodal learners who are comfortable with more than one style. We are told that, not surprisingly, journalists dominate in the reading/writing style, architects dominate in visual learning preferences, and most elite athletes are kinesthetic in their learning.

| | |
|---|---|
| **Visual** | Maps, graphics, charts, patterns, shapes. Could equally be called 'Graphics'. Does not include photos or videos. |
| **Auditory** | Heard or spoken. Sometimes speak before they sort their ideas. May repeat what has been said or ask a question that has been asked, to express in their own words. |
| **Reading, writing** | Words. Very common style. |
| **Kinisthetic** | Learning through experience and practice. Includes demonstrations, simulations, videos, movies, as well as case studies, practice and applications. |

**Table 4.1** VARK learning styles

ii. You can see more details and take the VARK test at https://vark-learn.com

Learning styles can potentially differ across domains; we may have dominant learning styles in one aspect of our lives, such as at work, that differ from how we might learn a sport. This is much more likely if we are multimodal learners.

It is probably obvious that knowing what kind of learner we are can make a real difference to how we perform. Being more aware of how we seek out ways to learn, and how we wish to receive information from others, can make the whole process so much less demanding and more successful. A large part of this is optimising how we and the people around us communicate with each other to enhance mutual understanding. So while learning how we learn may be part of metacognition, self-awareness, it is also a step forward in being self-effective through communicating. It can influence how we communicate with others, and how we ask them to communicate in return.

# 5

# Success Does Not Equal Perfect

*Le mieux est l'ennemi du bien.*
The perfect is the enemy of the good.

**Voltaire**

'Perfect'. The perfect experience. The perfect holiday. The perfect meal. The perfect day. The perfect weather. We all use the word freely to describe a great experience, even though we know that really, nothing is ever absolutely perfect. The point is, it doesn't need to be in order to be great. The same applies to performance. Nobody is perfect; it is an unattainable goal. Ask Tiger Woods, or Roger Federer, or any other great performer in any other sphere. These people show that perfection is not a key to high performance. They may aim for it, but they know they will not attain it.

Admittedly, some highly successful people are indeed perfectionists, but they have learned to channel that trait successfully. They have learned the art of mastery: achieving extremely high skills or attaining a comprehensive knowledge relating to a specific thing. Seeking mastery is not seeking perfection. Striving to do something better, striving for excellence, and being committed are all positive traits, but expecting 'perfect' outcomes will only leave us disappointed and will get in the way of performing well. Trying to perfect something is also inefficient; if we spend vast amounts of time focusing on one thing, we will neglect the other important elements that really count; it will cripple our progress, and indeed some people are paralysed by perfectionism. Fearing that something we do won't be perfect can stop us from performing well and creates performance anxiety; and there is strong evidence that perfectionism can lead to unhappiness and health issues, especially relating to mental health. 'My life has been nothing but a failure,' perfectionist Claude Monet once said. How terribly sad that he did not experience personal fulfilment from the beauty he created.

The emphasis on achieving perfection is increasing in our society. Research has shown that younger generations are increasingly demanding of themselves; characteristics of perfectionism are statistically on the rise, and are linked to mental health issues including anxiety and depression.[36]

Perfectionism is a trait that is described as '*having unrealistically high expectations and overly critical self-evaluations*'.[37] There is a big difference between being conscientious and motivated (good) and being a perfectionist (not so good). Recognising perfectionism is part of the process of learning to perform in a more fulfilling way. There are scales that can measure this.[38] Once perfectionism has been recognised, it can be channelled into something more productive, beginning with making small changes in the way the person thinks and how they behave. This is not threatening to the perfectionist's high standards; it is just a more successful way of gaining fulfilment from the effort. While some see this as transforming the perfectionist into a 'successful imperfectionist', this term has a negative connotation in relation to performance. A more positive approach is to focus on a transition to a 'pragmatic perfectionist' through realistic thinking, defining success, obtaining feedback rather than relying on one's own, seeing the bigger picture and the implications of actions, and last but not least, maintaining a sense of humour.

PART 2

# THE SIX KEYS

# 6

# Passion for the Purpose

*Your reason and your passion are the rudder and the sails of your seafaring soul. If either your sails or your rudder be broken, you can but toss and drift, or else be held at a standstill in midseas.*

**Kahlil Gibran**

## It All Starts with Passion

In their paper on passion and personality, Balon and colleagues[39] highlight a French maxim, '*La sagesse fait durer, les passions font vivre*', which translates to: 'Wisdom lengthens life, but passions make us live'.[40] They go on to highlight how throughout history, passion has been the driving force behind human progress, a source of strength and empowerment and leading to great achievements.[41] Such insights stem from the 1990s, when positive psychology arrived on the scene of psychology research and development.[42] It has dramatically advanced our insights into the importance of positivity to vitality, self-effectiveness, and performance.

Part of the positive psychology movement is passion, which can have a profound impact on our psychology, our happiness, and our function, and so it deserves its place in this book as the first Key. In life, we find things we enjoy largely through trial and error, and within that group of things, some become particularly meaningful to us and we become 'bonded' to them. That is what passion is, defined as a strong inclination towards a self-defining activity (or object) that one likes (or even loves), finds important and meaningful, and in which one invests time and energy.[43] It's a hunger for something. Passion entails a special relationship with an activity that one likes or loves, and to be a passion it is essential that this activity be meaningful for the person and part of one's identity.[44] It is this internalization, this link to our identity, that makes passion so important to our lives and our performances. So rather than being someone who is dedicated to being a great golfer, who practices deliberately and shows long-term commitment, when they become passionate about it, they become a Golfer, or similarly, someone might move from playing the piano to being a Pianist. And of course, in the context of this whole book, and performing in life in a fulfilling way, we hope to move from performing, to being a Performer.

There are seven core elements of passion.[45] First, passion relates to a specific activity, as opposed to a generalized passion for everything and anything. Second, passion encapsulates a profound and enduring love of that activity. Third, passion develops only towards activities that are personally valued or meaningful. Fourth, passion is associated with motivation. Fifth, passion emerges when activities become self-defining and part of one's identity. Sixth, passion encompasses high levels of psychological energy, effort, and persistence. Seventh, passion takes a dualistic form, which means it is a double-edged sword that can result in positive or negative outcomes.

This 'double-edged sword' of passion (the 'duality model') means there are two principal types: harmonious passion and obsessive passion. Both forms involve an investment of personal energy and time, but the outcomes can be very different, depending on the type.

The positive form of passion, **harmonious passion**, applies to engagement in activities that we love and which give us pleasure both throughout the activity and once we complete it. When we participate in an activity that brings us harmonious passion, we are more engaged,

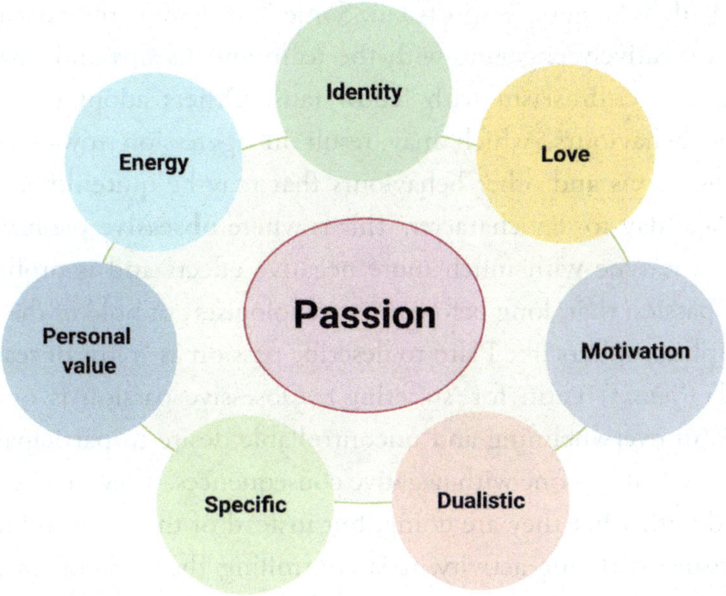


**Figure 6.1** Features of passion.

concentrate at a greater level, and feel happier, which in turn benefits other aspects of life. For example, a study of 277 recreational cyclists showed a direct correlation between their harmonious passion for the activity and their performance at work.[46] The evidence indicates that harmonious passion is positively correlated with vitality,[47] positive mood,[48] pursuing set goals, deliberate practice,[49] and maintenance of control over the activity,[50] amongst other positive behaviours. So possessing harmonious passion about something enhances that individual's performance. It therefore makes sense for those who support that individual (e.g., their employer) to encourage the individual in that activity. Passionate workforces are more effective and creative[51] and respond better to challenging situations.[52] In workplaces where there is empowering leadership – i.e., where the leaders create an atmosphere of positivity and motivate employees to be autonomous and more self-effective – this also enhances those employees' passion for the work.[53]

Eric Cantona said, 'If you have only one passion in life... and you pursue it to the exclusion of all other things, this becomes dangerous'. It is no secret that some things that you love can be good for you and some can be bad. Take being a sports fan. Some fans demonstrate harmonious passion, positively engaging with the team and its ups and downs and sharing that enthusiasm with fellow fans. Others adopt maladaptive, negative behaviours, which may result in aggression towards fans of opposing teams and other behaviours that may be quite different from their usual day-to-day character. This is where **obsessive passion** comes in. It is the type with much more negative effects and is probably the type of passion that, long before the psychologists got hold of the subject, caused philosophers like Plato to describe passion as 'a loss of reason and control' ('*passio*', Latin for 'suffering'). Obsessive passion is one where there is an overwhelming and uncontrollable desire to participate in an activity, even if it is one with negative consequences. They may feel totally engaged with what they are doing, but instead of them controlling their relationship with the activity, it is controlling them. Another example is someone who loves playing poker, but the passion is obsessive and keeps them at the table long after they should have left, with potentially damaging consequences. Obsessive passion is associated with negative consequences including rumination,[54] impaired concentration,[55] negative mood state during activity engagement and when the individual is prevented from doing the activity,[56] and in sport, increased likelihood of injuries.[57] Harmonious passion is associated with life satisfaction – but obsessive passion is not.

## Building Passion

Some individuals exhibit higher passion levels in general than do others. For most, passion is most likely a positive (harmonious) experience rather than a negative (obsessive) one, but it is possible to develop both in relation to separate activities. Passion is not a personality trait, but nevertheless it can be influenced by certain traits and characteristics. Specifically, if we consider the Big Five Personality traits – Openness, Conscientiousness, Extraversion, Agreeableness and Neuroticism (OCEAN) – the first four are positively linked to harmonious passion.[58] Of these, *conscientiousness* plays a particularly strong role in performance, and is discussed later. One of the reasons why conscientiousness influences harmonious passion is through an increased ability to self-regulate behaviours, resulting in the

| FEATURES | HARMONIOUS PASSION | OBSESSIVE PASSION |
|---|---|---|
| Deliberate practice | ++ | + |
| Cognitive-emotional engagement | +++ | o |
| Life satisfaction | ++ | o |
| Vitality | ++ | o |
| Concentration | ++ | + |
| Flow | +++ | ++ |
| Self-esteem | + | – |
| Anxiety | – – | + |
| Rumination | o | +++ |
| Intrinsic motivation | +++ | ++ |
| Mastery | ++ | + |
| Regulation | +++ | ++ |
| Satisfaction of psychological need | ++ | + |
| Activity/life conflict | – | ++ |

**Table 6.1** Correlation between passion and other factors.

**+** = small **++** = moderate **+++** = large positive correlation
**–** = small negative correlation **– –** = moderate negative correlation
**o** = no correlation

ability to change behaviours to suit goals, and/or to disengage from those behaviours when necessary. Furthermore, those who successfully build harmonious passion often exhibit powers of perseverance. Obsessive passion, on the other hand, usually is associated with limited levels of both self-regulation and perseverance.[59] A low level of Agreeableness is associated with obsessive passion, but the other traits have no influence. Neuroticism has no link to either forms of passion. Hence, some associations do exist between passion and personality, but a host of other factors play a role.

Some lucky people develop a passion for what they do in life at a very early stage, and it drives them forward quickly. For most, though, passion in relation to an activity develops with time. Regardless of when it occurs, its development is largely influenced by learning experiences, positive mentorship, enhancement of autonomy, peer support, positive feedback, the immediate environment and factors that drive motivation, which will be discussed in the next chapter. Hence, passion can be built, and a focus on those factors that enhance the harmonious type can enhance the lives of individuals and the people around them. Furthermore, seeking to avoid obsessive passion, which can develop due to external pressures, lack of support, and loss of identity, is key.

## Key Messages:

- Passion relates to a specific activity and encapsulates a profound and enduring love of that activity that is personally valued.
- Passion is associated with motivation and encompasses high levels of psychological energy, effort, and persistence.
- Passion is part of a person's identity.
- Harmonious passion is a significant positive influence on health, well-being, and performance.
- Passion can be built through positive learning experiences, environments, support, and mentorship.
- Obsessive passion is a risk.

# 7

# Perseverance

*Success is no accident. It is hard work, perseverance, learning, studying, sacrifice, and most of all, love of what you are doing or learning to do.*

**Pele**

No matter how passionate we are about an activity and the pursuit of a goal, we all need powers of perseverance to succeed. Perseverance means 'continued effort to do or achieve something despite difficulties, failure, or opposition'.[60] It is, in essence, sustained persistence. Without it, learning, mastery, and expertise are not achieved. It requires self-discipline, self-regulation, and commitment to achieving goals that may take considerable time and effort to attain, often under circumstances that deplete mental, emotional, and physical resources.

Perseverance accounts for many successes. We would not have the lightbulb if Thomas Edison had not persevered even after thousands of attempts did not succeed; many Wimbledon champions would not have won without persevering when their opponents were on match point; we would not have seen many industrial advances if Henry Ford had not persevered after a number of bankruptcies; Vincent Van Gogh continued to paint prolifically even though he had sold only one painting (and that was to a friend); Larry Page and Sergey Brin showed great powers of perseverance in getting financial support to start Google and to take it from a 7.8% share of the search-engine market to dominating the field and becoming a household name years later. Then there are the great explorers like Ernest Shackleton, who even if ultimately unsuccessful in achieving an improbable goal, still achieved the unimaginable beforehand, through leadership, planning, and especially perseverance.

## A Note on 'Grit'

Those who read widely about human performance will be familiar with the concept of 'grit', proposed by one group in 2007 to be a personality trait that reflects 'perseverance and passion for long-term goals', and *the* thing that predicts achievement, especially academic achievement.[61] The proposal became popular, and for this reason it is mentioned here. Many experts though have contested this claim, demonstrating that 'grit' is an over-simplification, and only a weak predictor of performance and success, and at best may reflect some aspects of conscientiousness, passion, and perseverance.[62] Attractive as it may be to integrate different important elements of performance into one term, grit scales that are used do not give clear insights into these separate elements, and there is no evidence that grit as a single entity predicts success.[63] For example, as with all Keys to performance, perseverance and passion influence each other. Both have impacts on performance and reaching goals that are independent of one another but are greatest when passion and perseverance are both high. It is known that passion enhances perseverance, probably through a heightened intensity of focus on the task(s). That's not too surprising – if we love what we do, we are more likely to persevere.

A number of the elements discussed throughout this book are related to perseverance: dealing with setbacks, following learning curves, having a plan, coping with stress, maintaining self-belief, sticking with good habits, etc. You will also see how perseverance is influenced by the other Keys, including conscientiousness and self-efficacy. Passion also has a large influence, but note that it differs from motivation, which is a key component of perseverance. While passion is the love for something, motivation is the trigger to actions that keep the process going.

## Motivation

Motivation means 'the internal and/or external forces that produce the initiation, direction, intensity and persistence of behaviour'.[64] It is the machine that keeps us going, the driving force behind our actions that helps us to persevere towards goals that we are (hopefully) passionate about.

We start with **activation**, the initial trigger that gets us going. An example is the early alarm bell that signals it's time to get up and head for that exercise session before work. It was easy enough to have made the plan towards a fitness goal from our sofa one evening, and is often more manageable to motivate ourselves during those summer months when it is light when we wake up and the birds are singing, but in those dark cold winter months, motivation often wanes. Finding the right motivational steps that activate the process is the trick. Those triggers will often change during a performance journey, even if the goal remains the same, and Mark Twain was right in this respect when he said, '*The first step is to take one*'.

It's smart to have some form of motivating cue that gets us going on those dark mornings, that one thing that makes us perform the first action to get the ball rolling in the right direction. That might be simply switching on the light to see some running shoes sitting by the bed, or having motivating music to flick the switch into 'get moving' mode. Having a clear direction is a keystone in staying motivated to persevere, and that direction – the strategy – must be clear, acting as signposts along the journey. The direction and the signposts should be reviewed regularly and changed according to experience, progress and circumstances. Once the two initial parts of motivation are harnessed, perseverance and maintenance become so much easier.

**Activation → Direction → Perseverance**

**Figure 7.1** Components of motivation.

When we are particularly passionate about something it is easier to stay motivated than when that passion is not as strong. A simple example relates to those administrative tasks we address on a day-to-day basis that we frequently put off because we find them tedious. Linking them to the goals we are more passionate about helps us to find the necessary motivation to do them, and even to find some bonding with the process. As you read further through this book you will see how the whole process of motivation and perseverance is made easier not just by building passion but through optimising the other Keys too: self-awareness of how we respond to the prospect of specific tasks and motivational triggers; self-efficacy helps us make necessary changes; planning, habits, and timing what we do and when (aided by conscientiousness and our chronobiology); and of course possessing energy and positivity (vitality).

## Intrinsic and Extrinsic Motivation

So, back to more about motivation in its own right. Motivation is partly based on an individual's needs, typically described according to five levels (Maslow's Hierarchy), with the highest level potentially having the greatest impact.[65] Motivation itself can be classified as either intrinsic or extrinsic. **Intrinsic motivation** is that which is performed for the pleasure and satisfaction of performing the behaviour itself, because they are curious, enjoy learning, and/or find the activity challenging and satisfying.[66] Intrinsic motivation is a life-long psychological and personal growth function. **Extrinsic motivation** is where the behaviour is performed for some form of externally driven reward (e.g., financial) or to avoid punishment/negative consequences.[67]

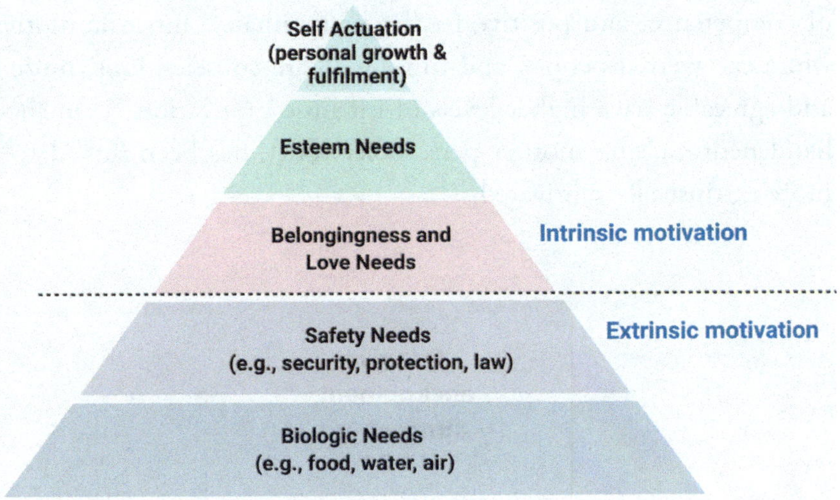


**Figure 7.2** Motivation and the hierarchy of needs.

It was previously thought that the most motivated people would be those with high intrinsic and extrinsic levels, but in fact we now know that extrinsic motivation results in a decrease in intrinsic motivation, due to a loss of autonomy for the individual; he or she no longer has control of the 'reward'.[68] This does not mean that financial rewards should be lightened nor their role underestimated, but rather that paying someone well may only initiate engagement, not sustain it. Intrinsic motivation stems from our innate desires to be 'self-determined', autonomous,[69] and effective,[70] and extrinsic motivations – since driven by others – can be perceived as a threat to those desires. You will soon see why self-efficacy has a role here, as it reflects our belief in our abilities to control our destiny. In essence, the more a task is autonomous, driven by a person's own free will, the greater the intrinsic motivation and the more positive the outcomes. This has been found to apply to a range of activities and aspects of life, including relationships, education, sport and exercise, and healthy ageing.[71] However, intrinsic motivation does not necessarily happen automatically; it can be negatively or positively impacted, for example by environments and cultures, peer pressure, sense of competence, and feedback. Positive, supportive environments and philosophies, strong peer support, a sense of competence, and positive feedback all enhance intrinsic motivation. More extraverted people, and those who are conscientious, more open, and agreeable have higher levels of intrinsic motivation.[72] On the other hand neuroticism (another personality trait), has been linked to being more extrinsically motivated.

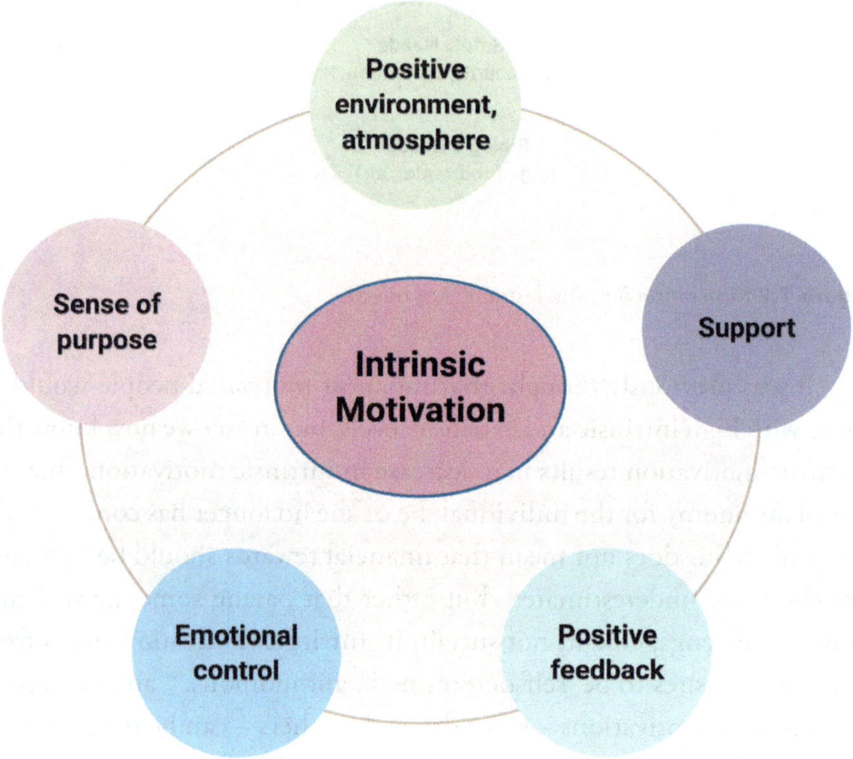


**Figure 7.3** Factors that influence intrinsic motivation.

The neuroscience of motivation is still being teased out. However, we know that intrinsic motivation includes complex cognitive, emotional, and behavioural elements that are driven by a number of signals within the brain and across its circuits. Central to this is dopamine, which is a chemical released in the brain that plays a role in habit formation and is often called the 'pleasure chemical' because it is associated with a sense of reward, for example when a craving is satisfied. It is also associated with enhanced mood, flexibility of thinking, creativity, curiosity, and persistence/perseverance Research has shown that those with higher capacities for intrinsic motivation have more receptors for dopamine in their brains,[73] and other studies using fMRI, PET scanning, and EEG show an association between dopamine signalling and motivation.[74]

Enlightened organisations that are great employers seek to fulfil and motivate their workforce through positive team cultures, an emphasis on personal development and fulfilment, a sense of purpose in the organisation and beyond, and creating great environments to work in. As this book is being written, much of the world has worked from home for many months due to the Covid-19 pandemic. Finding new ways to support and motivate employees in this new era is a challenge but a necessity. Expertise in performance-based sciences, health and well-being initiatives, and innovative technologies undoubtedly will be key.

# 8

# Conscientiousness

*I daily examine myself on three points: In planning for others, have I failed in conscientiousness? In intercourse with friends, have I been insincere? And have I failed to practice what I have been taught?*

**Confucius**

Much is made of personality traits in relation to human performance, and in particular the 'Big Five' personality types: Openness, Conscientiousness, Agreeableness, Extraversion, and Neuroticism (OCEAN). However, there is scant evidence that any of them truly predict outcomes, *except* for conscientiousness. Conscientiousness means being goal orientated, disciplined, organised, and diligent. It is considered a personality trait influenced by 'nature and nurture', and although up to 44% may be determined by our genetics,[75] the rest is influenced by environment, upbringing, and training. Conscientiousness is linked to high agreeableness and low levels of extraversion, neuroticism, and openness.[76] Although it is partly ingrained, we can optimise it by training specific components

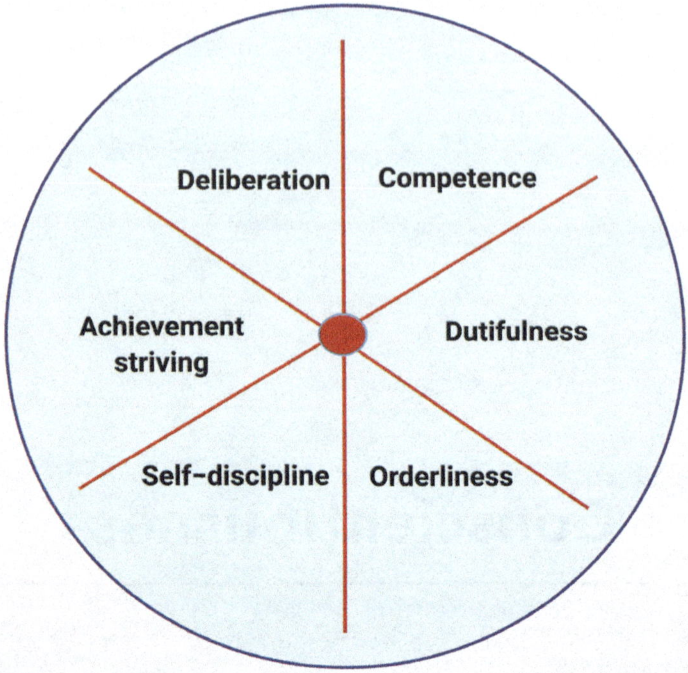


**Figure 8.1** Features of conscientiousness.

through focused attention on habits and planning, starting, for example, with developing discipline in performing one or a few things.

There are six principal facets of conscientiousness: orderliness, dutifulness, achievement striving, self-discipline, deliberation, and competence. For ease, particularly in relation to assessment, some simply describe conscientiousness in two domains: order and industriousness. Although it is frequently assumed that discipline and self-regulation are dominant in conscientiousness, there is evidence that the trait is also associated with flexibility and the ability to adapt to changing environmental contingencies and task demands.[77] So 'being disciplined enough to be adaptable' may be a way of viewing it.

Conscientiousness is linked to executive function, which you will recall are the mental processes that include focus, planning, working memory, self-regulation, and taking specific actions.

Conscientiousness has a significant impact on many aspects of daily living. It is linked to well-being and stands out as a 'singularly striking

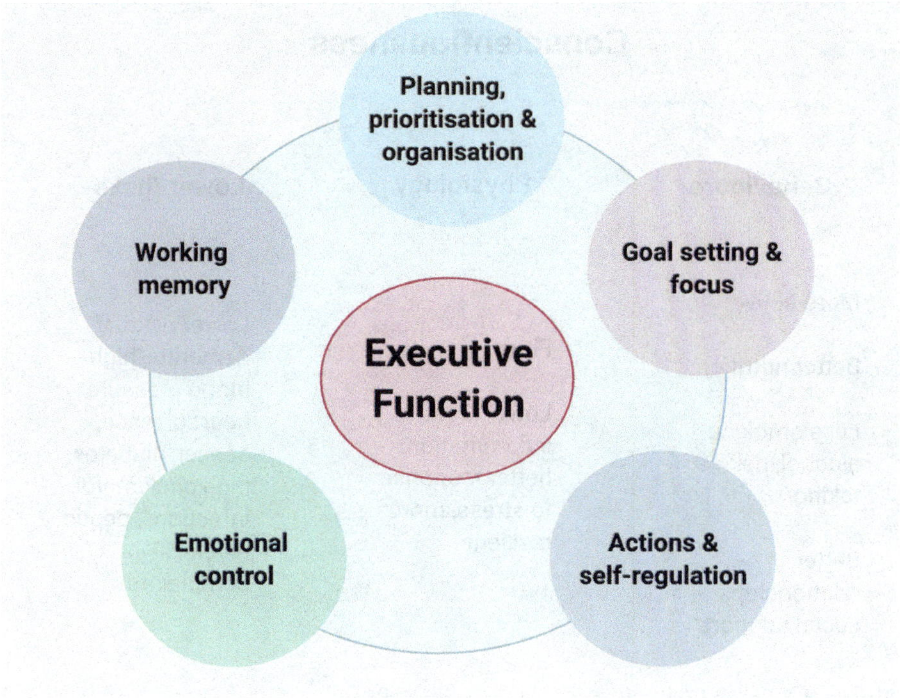


**Figure 8.2** Components of executive function.

predictor of health throughout life'.[78] It is associated with reduced risk for many illnesses [79] and with positive biomarkers of health [80]. It is also negatively associated with mortality.[81] Research suggests that conscientious people have lower cortisol (stress hormone) levels than others. A study in 2017 analysed a three-centimeter sample of hair from over 2,000 subjects, allowing a measure of three months' worth of cortisol accumulation, along with measurement of lifestyle behaviours and personality traits.[82] The lower cortisol levels and better lifestyles were seen in those with higher conscientiousness, but seemingly were not driven simply by lifestyle, and so most likely conscientious people have different responses to stress that may be inborn or developed through training, or both.

Conscientiousness is also linked to better academic, job and workplace performance, and career success.[83] In sport, successful athletes are more likely to have strong levels of conscientiousness,[84] particularly in individual sports. In team sports, those with higher conscientiousness levels are more likely to be leaders and captains.[85] Conscientious people

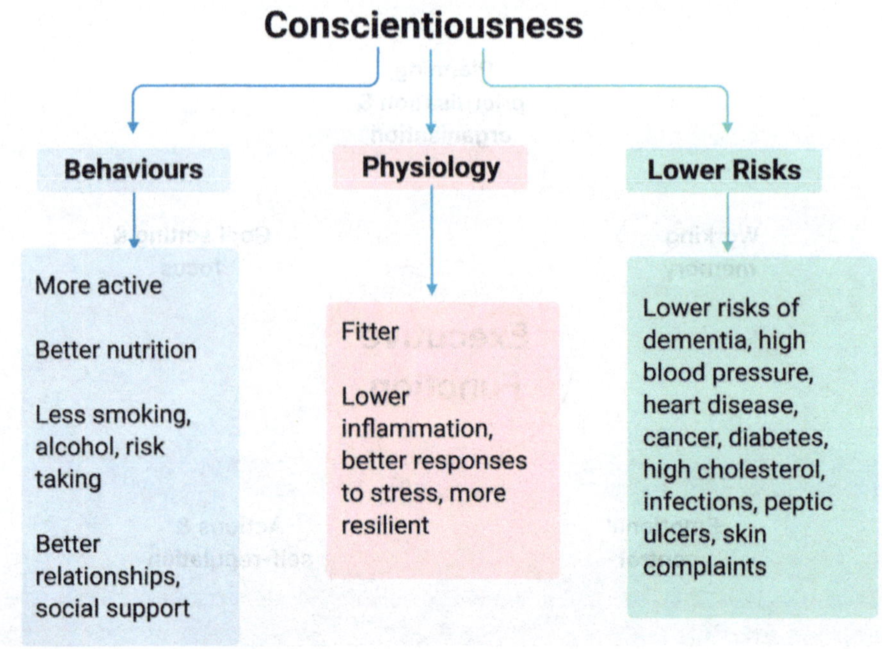


**Figure 8.3** Some health benefits of conscientiousness.

tend to be competitive and motivated to excel and improve their skills,[86] and in general are more responsive to training.[87] However, there are some less good associations too; conscientiousness can be associated with a higher tendency to procrastinate, greater chance of burnout,[88] and a higher tendency to perfectionism.[89]

Given all that has been said above, it should not be surprising that conscientiousness is a step towards a healthier, longer, and happier life. This has been shown to be the case across diverse populations and different age groups, and it is independent of intelligence. This effect on longevity is significant, and in fact has been shown to have three times the size of the effect of socioeconomic status.[90]

## Measuring Conscientiousness

Conscientiousness is often evaluated in combination with other personality traits, but there are a number of validated tools in scientific papers to assess it separately.[91] There are also a range of scores available for a price online, which are less transparent and hence probably best avoided. In essence it all boils down to how high or low the individual scores in the features listed in table 8.1.[92]

| High | Low |
| --- | --- |
| • Competent<br>• Organized<br>• Dutifulness<br>• Achievment striving<br>• Self-disciplined<br>• Deliberation | • Incompetent<br>• Disorganized<br>• Careless<br>• Procrastinates<br>• Indiscipline<br>• Impulsive |

**Table 8.1** Features of high and low levels of conscientiousness.

## Optimising Conscientiousness

The evidence suggests that making small changes in conscientiousness can have a significant impact on performance.[93] Just focusing on a few things will help, and this can be self-driven and/or with the support of a mentor or coach, often as part of a wider performance programme. Making some changes does require some motivation, discipline, and effort, and the latter two of these are what people who have low levels of conscientiousness lack. Planning schedules in advance, using an understanding of chronobiology to help us to schedule when we perform certain tasks (discussed later in chapter 12), setting reminders on our mobile phones, tidying/organising work areas – these are all examples of steps that can assist. **Mindfulness** training can be helpful in enhancing conscientiousness, and a process called 'cognitive remediation' may also be beneficial, although not yet formally studied specifically relating to conscientiousness. It is a tool used to enhance executive functions, where the user works through a series of cognitive exercises and video games, with the resulting improvement in executive functions also having positive effects on conscientiousness.

*It takes as much energy to wish as it does to plan.*

**Eleanor Roosevelt**

## Habits

*First we make our habits, then our habits make us.*

**John Dryden**

Our habits in life can often have significant consequences, and they are influenced by our conscientiousness. A habit is *'a routine or practice performed regularly, an automatic response to a specific situation'*. Many habits are autopilot, 'no constant control required by the operator'. Habits by definition are engrained behaviours, performed subconsciously, usually in response to a specific cue or context. They take little effort unless, of course, we want to change them; *then* it can become challenging. Habits dominate our success and failure in achieving specific goals, but how are habits are formed, and how do we de-programme and re-programme the ones we want to change? This is where conscientiousness comes in, because being conscientious helps – *a lot*. Simply put, conscientious people tend to build, maintain and change habits more successfully, and it is those habits that lead to the benefits in physiology, vitality, and performance. Conscientious people are also better at altering their habits when needed.

### How Habits Are Formed

Habits are formed as a result of multiple signalling processes in our brains. Typically, the process starts by making a conscious decision to do something; it sets a goal. For example, putting our seatbelt on when we get in the car. That decision-making centre is in the pre-frontal cortex of the brain. As we repeat the behaviour – every time we get into the car, we put our seatbelt on – another part of the brain, the striatum in the basal ganglia, starts to take over. An automated loop forms and the behaviour becomes a habit and is subconscious. The decision-making centre is then freed up to focus on other things. The striatum is an area that is rich in dopamine, the pleasure-seeking chemical that drives the brain's reward pathway, which helps to embed the habit in the brain's wiring. Sometimes we will be aware of that reward, but the more times you repeat the habit the less apparent that reward might be. An example would be after dinner

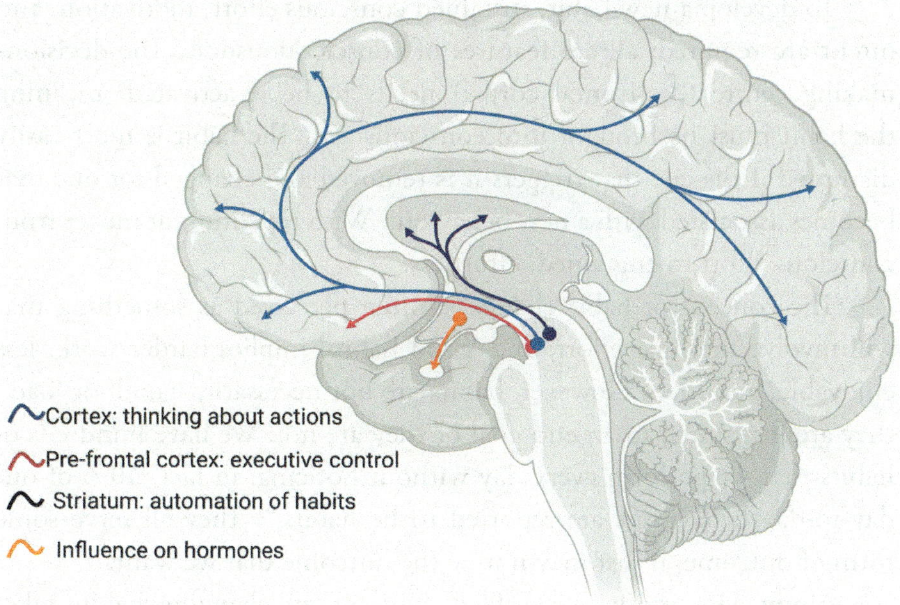


**Figure 8.4** Dopamine pathways in the brain serve many different areas and processes.

we decide to have a rich dessert. At first it's amazing, so we start having one every night after dinner, and it becomes a habit. With time, we notice the pleasure of eating it less.

Habits typically involve four steps: the cue, the craving, the response (behaviour), and the reward (the habit loop).[94] The cue represents a certain context, situation, or other prompt that sometimes triggers a conscious craving/desire to do something, and the response follows. Sometimes the cue just triggers a subconscious behaviour, without a craving. For example, putting on a seat belt (action/behaviour) after getting into the car (cue), or smokers having a cigarette (action) after eating dinner or with a cup of coffee (cue). In the smoking example, there is a craving after the cue, a conscious desire, a drive to act out the behaviour, and that craving varies between habits. There also is the conscious reward that may be experienced once the behaviour has been performed, often in the form of pleasure gained from the action. But as mentioned earlier, with some habits, the reward may not be noticed. Locking the front door on leaving the house, tying our shoelaces after putting on our shoes, and so on.

To develop a new habit, sustained conscious effort, motivation, and intent are required; all are features of conscientiousness. The decision-making centre (pre-frontal cortex) needs to be re-activated, meaning the habit must be brought into consciousness. The habit is most easily disrupted if the cue that triggers it is removed and changed for one that becomes associated with a new behaviour. With repetition, it moves from conscious effort to engrained, effortless.

The concept of habit change is often perceived as something that will involve tiresome effort; and 'good habits' implies harder work, less enjoyable, a burden. However, habits are not necessarily 'good' or 'bad', they are just suited to an end goal or they are not. We have hundreds of habits that we perform every day without noticing; in fact, 40% of our day-to-day behaviours are reported to be habits.[95] They all serve some form of outcome; it just may not be the outcome that we want.

Along with motivation, effort, and intent, changing habits takes time. It is often said that developing a new habit, or changing one, takes 21 days, but this is a myth. How long it takes depends on the habit,

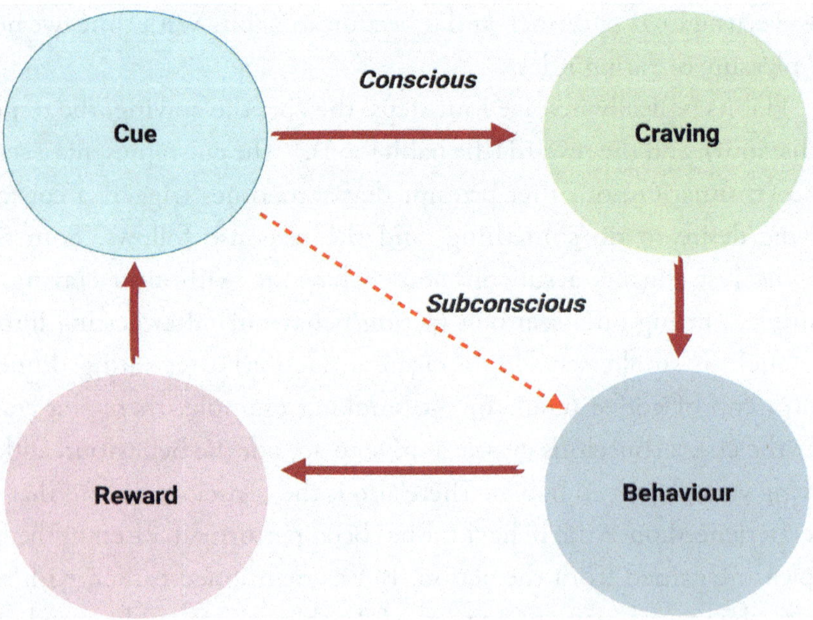


**Figure 8.5** The habit loop.

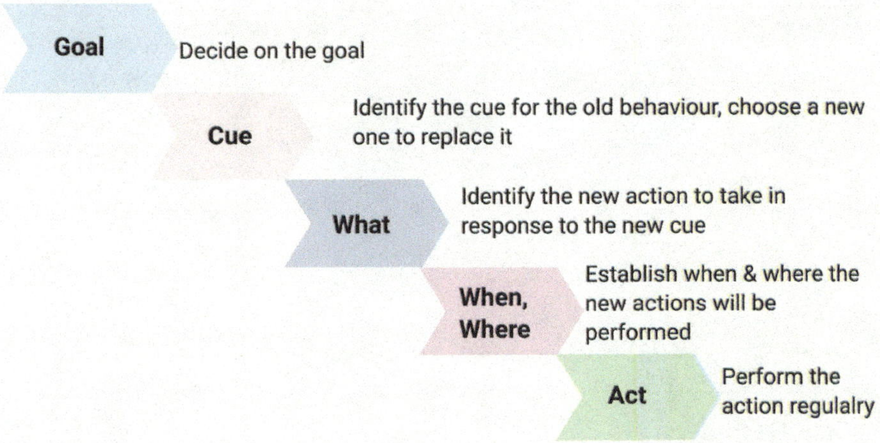


**Figure 8.6** Steps towards creating a new habit

the person, and the circumstances. Research has indicated it can take anywhere from 18 to 254 days to change an eating, drinking, or activity habit.[96] The more the new habit is practiced, the quicker it becomes 'wired' into the brain. One study has suggested that those who take up a new exercise programme are more likely to be successful in establishing it as a habit if they engage in it at least four times per week for the first six weeks. Also, the simpler the regime and the more enjoyable it is, the more likely it will become a sustained behaviour across time.[97] No surprises there.

Changing one habit can have an impact on other elements. For example, altering something associated with our health-related routines such as changing to eating an evening meal earlier → better sleep; metabolism improves → we wake more energised; energy balance improves → we become more active → we make healthier choices → we lose some weight… etc.

# 9

# Self-Efficacy

*Believe*

What feature unites Nelson Mandela, Roger Federer, Steven Hawking, Dolly Parton, Tiger Woods, and Albert Einstein (amongst others)? Self-efficacy. Why do some top sportsmen and women seem to be able to turn around a match when they appear to be beaten? Self-efficacy. Why do some people cope so well in unexpected crises? Self-efficacy.

Self-efficacy means our self-belief, the 'power of believing you can',[98] and how we adapt, self-manage, and self-regulate to achieve a goal.[99] It is critical to vitality and performance. It dominates how we behave and how we process challenges, and it can be the difference between success and failure. Self-efficacy plays a major part in daily functioning, affecting thinking and decision making and a person's ability to control their personal destiny.[100] It is *not* about inborn 'talent'; it is *not* a personality trait; and it is *not* the same as self-esteem, which means how we feel about ourselves and our beliefs – how much we *like* ourselves. Self-efficacy is built through learning and experiences and how we mentally process and reflect on these. There is a really good reason why our academic reading on this subject should start with two iconic texts: *Oh, the Places You'll Go!* by Dr Seuss,[101] and *The Little Engine that Could*, by Watty Piper.[102] There's also a very good reason why children should read (or be read) these books when young, since self-efficacy develops from childhood and continues to evolve throughout our lives.

How does self-efficacy make such a big impact? It's fairly straightforward: those who are more self-effective set higher goals, are more likely to self-motivate, are more likely to put in the effort, problem solve, be positive and optimistic, and persevere.[103] They are simply more likely to perform well. Having high self-efficacy means we are more likely to adapt well to new situations, have a proactive 'can-do' attitude, stay motivated, deal better with stress, take on more challenging tasks, have more optimistic outlooks, stick to our goals, and achieve better satisfaction with life.[104] Not surprisingly, there is some overlap with the other Key Characteristics of performing well, especially conscientiousness and perseverance.

Research has shown that self-efficacy has relevance across most domains in life; in studying, at work, at home, in relation to our health, and in our satisfaction with life. Those with higher self-efficacy are more likely to be employed, are in much better heath, and have greater life-satisfaction than those with lower self-efficacy.

Self-efficacy can be considered in a general context, encompassing how people function and their coping skills in life in general. It may also relate to very specific beliefs about their abilities to coordinate skills and abilities to attain very specific goals, in a specific area, and under specific circumstances. Hence the extent of one's self-efficacy can be different across different domains, higher in some elements of life than in others. An example would be having very high academic self-efficacy but much lower self-efficacy in regulation of behaviours such as nutrition and exercise. We all know people whom we wonder how they can be so successful in some things and disastrous in others.

*If I have the belief that I can do it, I shall surely acquire the capacity to do it even if I may not have it at the beginning.*

**Mahatma Gandhi**

## Self-Efficacy and Vitality

In essence, self-efficacy is largely about positive psychology, which you will have noted from the introduction is an important part of vitality, and this is one of the many reasons why self-effectiveness is so important to performance. If we are more self-effective. we are more likely to have positive health behaviours[105] and be happy and healthy, and vice versa. Self-efficacy can also influence biological processes such as enhancing physiological responses to stress and immune function.[106]

Self-efficacy is linked to better self-regulation, which is the way we regulate our thoughts, emotions, and behaviours to suit a goal, and in terms of health, that includes regulating behaviours relating to exercise, nutrition, stress management, addiction, and compliance with treatment and screening programmes.[107] People are more likely to stick with a programme and be regular exercisers,[108] and are also more likely to be successful in a weight loss programme,[109] if they have higher self-efficacy. On the flip side, low self-efficacy is associated with depression, anxiety, and helplessness. It also is associated with the ability to deal with stress, adversity, and pain, and the capacity to develop skills like mindfulness.[110]

### Self-Efficacy in Work and Careers

Studies have also shown consistent relationships between self-efficacy and work-based outcomes,[111] for example managerial performance,[112] skill acquisition,[113] managerial idea generating,[114] coping with career-related events,[115] adaptability to advanced technology,[116] adjustment to a new job,[117] and job-specific performance.[118] Occupational self-efficacy measured at career entry has a positive impact on salary and status three years later and a positive impact on salary change and career satisfaction seven years later.[119] Taking many studies of self-efficacy and work performance and evaluating them together in a meta-analysis, there is evidence that there is a significant correlation between the two, and that high self-efficacy results in a 28% gain in performance.[120] That's a big bang for your buck and outweighs anything demonstrated relating to the impact of personality traits on work-based performance, where there is still no clear systematic evidence for their effects.

### Self-Efficacy and Academic Performance

In academia, a student's perceived self-efficacy is a significant determinant of their academic achievement[121] and work-related performance.[122]

Gender differences have been demonstrated in elements of self-efficacy in a range of academic domains, and in life in general females are frequently found to have lower self-efficacy scores.[123] Academically, males are slightly more self-effective overall. Females display higher language and arts self-efficacy than males,[124] while males exhibit higher self-efficacy in the STEM subjects, economics, and social sciences.[125] The gender differences in self-efficacy are considered to relate to gender stereotypes in early development.[126] The presence of positive role models early in life is very influential in preventing this.

### Self-Efficacy and Sporting Performance

In sport, self-efficacy has been shown to positively influence performance across a range of pursuits, including tennis, diving, ski-jumping, and golf.[127]

What top sports star have you ever heard of succeeding without them believing in themselves? In marathon runners and triathletes, self-efficacy is associated with better performance; a remarkable 46% of the variance in finishing times in marathons has been reported to be explained by self-efficacy.[128] The influence of self-efficacy on sporting outcomes seems to be greatest in the early phase of a competitive event, although this may vary across sports and athletes.[129]

Recent literature has provided findings to show how self-efficacy can determine effort, persistence, and performance in exercise. In one study that examined simple hand grip (a significant health predictor, by the way), self-efficacy strongly positively influenced the ability to sustain longer periods of gripping.[130] The association between goal orientation, self-esteem, perceived ability, effort, commitment, exertion, feedback tolerance, and process/outcome measures has also been examined. Self-efficacy was shown to predict the length at which an individual can put forth effort and withstand discomfort.[131] In a computer-simulated running task, self-efficacy and task-specific psychological states accounted for 63 to 68% of the performance variance, representing a dramatic impact.

There is one caveat about self-efficacy and its impact on performance. In some with extreme self-efficacy, it can spill into being so over-confident that there is a lack of proper preparation, little motivation, and potential underperformance as a result.

## Measuring Self-Efficacy

There are two approaches to assessing self-efficacy; both are simple, and both involve self-report. One is to examine it in general, and the other is to examine it in relation to a specific goal. There are a number of validated self-report scales for general self-efficacy, and they address the individual's perceived ability to deal with challenges, complete complex tasks, and achieve goals. Over the years these have become more simplified, because simple scores (thankfully) seem to reflect self-efficacy very well.[iii]

Drawing from such general scales, goal-specific self-efficacy can be customised to assess it in relation to specific situations where performing a task to achieve a goal might become difficult (see the box below). It seems a simple thing to assess, but of course the challenge is then to address ways of improving it if needed.

In [*this situation*] when facing this task, I am certain that I will accomplish it.

- ☐ Strongly disagree
- ☐ Disagree
- ☐ Neither agree nor disagree
- ☐ Agree
- ☐ Strongly agree

iii. The Stanford University SPARQtools self-efficacy scale is an example of an easy-to-use test. You can find it at http://sparqtools.org/mobility-measure/new-general-self-efficacy-scale.

## Building Self-Efficacy

Clearly, self-efficacy is important to all of us, both in our personal and our professional lives. We are all faced with adapting to new circumstances and learning new skills, coping with significant pressures, remaining positive and acting proactively; and to do this and perform well in the process, self-efficacy is key.[132] Self-efficacy can and should be built from a young age, and is built through just a few key elements: having the right support, learning through experiences, role modelling, visualisation techniques, and very importantly, enhancing vitality (illustrated in figure 9.1 and table 9.1).

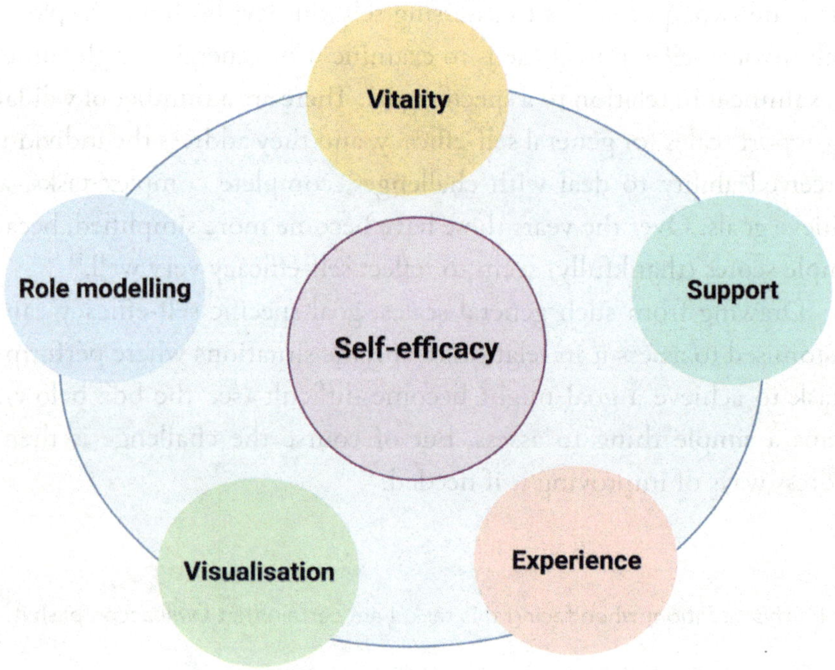


**Figure 9.1** Factors that influence self-efficacy.

| Factor | Tips |
|---|---|
| **Personal experience** | Success breeds success. When an individual has performed a task successfully, it is easier the next time. The converse is also true; when there is 'failure', then this becomes more likely the next time. Experiential learning and deliberate practice are central components to improving outcomes. |
| **Vicarious experience and role modelling** | Success by those whom the individual sees as similar to themself and role models, enhances their self-efficacy. So the individual should identify who those people are and keep them in their focus. |
| **Visualisation, imagery** | Imagining a successful outcome, imagery, improves self-belief. Refining how to perform imagery comes with mindfulness training. |
| **Support** | Receiving coaching and encouragement improves self-effectiveness. It is needed to assist with deliberate practice. |
| **Vitality** | Feeling good mentally and physically positively influences higher self-efficacy – and vice versa. |

**Table 9.1** Steps towards optimising self-efficacy.

Any programme that aims to build self-efficacy must build on these stepping stones. The importance of support must be emphasised: a coach and/or mentor helps to formalise the process, to develop imagery skills, identify role models, and assist in reflection on personal and vicarious experiences. Across many settings, creating challenges to allow personal development is part of the way self-efficacy can be developed, but exceeding a person's capacity and/or excessive emotional strain can have detrimental effects.[133]

As self-efficacy builds, it becomes easier to deal with challenges. When we are faced with a new, challenging situation in which we have no personal experience of the task(s) involved, if we can remember seeing it being dealt with by someone else (a role model), we have a mental image of their performance (imagery), and we can often identify someone who can provide support. These steps enhance our self-belief, and our ability to execute the behaviours needed to respond to the challenge. That's self-efficacy.

**Key Messages:**

- Self-efficacy means our self-belief, the 'power of believing you can', and how we adapt, self-manage, and self-regulate to achieve a goal.
- Self-efficacy plays a major role in our health and well-being and in our academic, professional, and sporting performances.
- Self-efficacy can be built from a young age with adequate training and techniques, learning and experience, support, mentorship, role modelling, and energy.

# 10

# Self-Awareness

*Know thyself*

**Ancient Greek aphorism**

It is all very well for the Ancient Greeks who came up with this phrase, but in this era of societal expectation, socioeconomic pressures, the culture of achievement, and living life on autopilot at a million miles an hour, 'knowing thyself' isn't so easy. Knowing thyself means self-awareness. Long after the Greeks highlighted the concept, philosophers continued to focus on what that means (and still do). '*Cogito, ergo sum*' ('I think therefore I am'), declared Descartes in his *Principles of Philosophy* (1644), a fundamental philosophical statement in relation to our recognition of our very existence. While we continue to cogitate on the meaning of self from a philosophical basis, much of the attention is now also given to its scientific basis.

In the context of human performance, self-awareness means recognising how our minds and bodies work, how we think, our emotions, how we learn, how we behave, and how we respond to our environments,

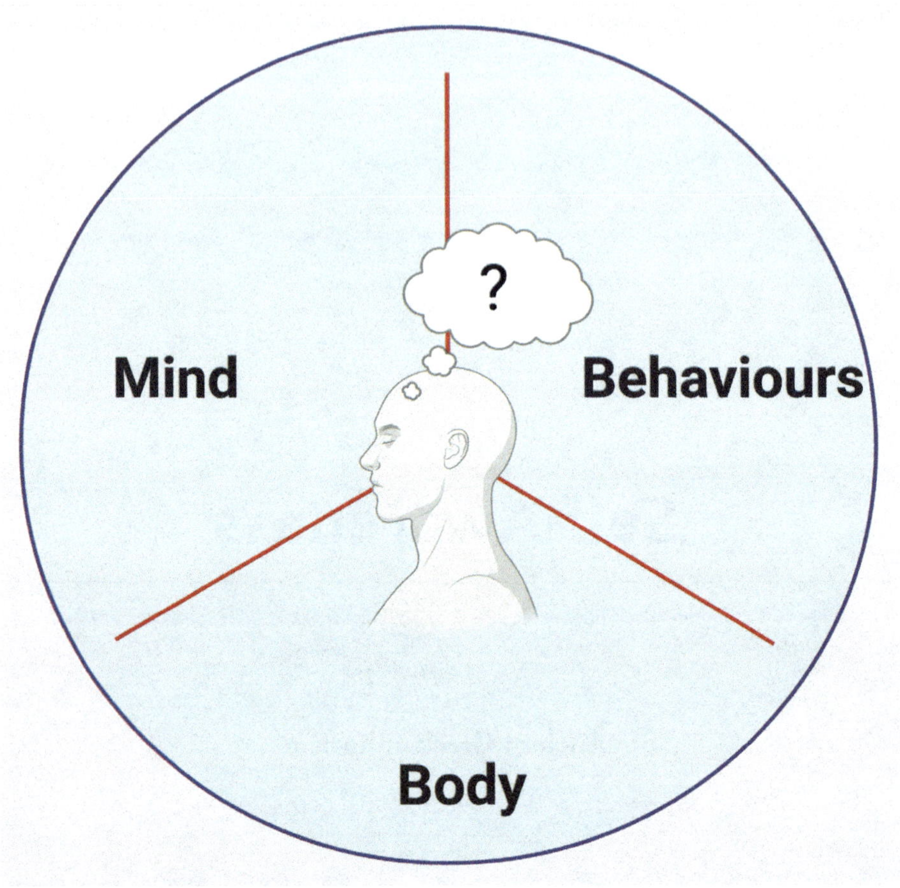


**Figure 10.1** Self-awareness: Conscious self-monitoring.

the people around us, challenges, and circumstances. It is partly 'thinking about how we think', also called 'metacognition', literally 'beyond' or 'higher order' thinking, 'conscious self-monitoring'.

The whole subject of self-awareness can make people uncomfortable, largely due to misconceptions about its meaning and what it entails. To many it represents a need to delve too deeply into who they are, or it involves admitting to negative attributes, or it's not cool, or it's too complex, or the process is too much trouble, or its all psycho-babble... None of these are true. As with most things, the first stage is to understand what self-awareness is, and then to take small steps to embrace it.

Whereas consciousness, being aware of our existence, does not require complex brains,[134] an advanced capacity for self-awareness does.

| Example | Benefit |
|---|---|
| **Insights into strengths and weaknesses** | Empowerment<br>Makes most performance journeys much easier |
| **Early detection of when we are stressed** | Channels stress towards positive responses<br>Protects health and well-being<br>Promotes better outcomes |
| **Body awareness** | Enhances health behaviours, fitness training, recovering from injury, illness<br>Helps with training a skill |
| **Awareness of how we learn** | Smooths the apprenticeship journey<br>Helps with training skills |
| **Awareness of how we like to communicate** | Improves relationships, smooths interactions, facilitates better outcomes |
| **Knowing what triggers specific behaviours** | Motivation, planning, perseverance |

**Table 10.1** Examples of some benefits of self-awareness.

Our ability as sophisticated animals to be self-aware is conferred by the size and architecture of our brains, and is mostly influenced by our cerebral cortex. As described earlier, this part of the human brain is big due to its convoluted design with its many folds and creases increasing it surface area. Other bits of the brain are important too, and this has been reinforced by the finding that even people with significant brain injuries affecting the cortex of the brain still have self-awareness.[135] Even though we have relatively small heads, the billions of nerve cells that interconnect make us potentially very sophisticated thinkers and part of that sophistication is being capable of self-awareness. We humans develop that self-awareness in the first year of our lives, and subsequently some develop it more than others, which is partly nature and partly nurture.

## Self-Awareness and Human Performance

A lot of people think they are self-aware, but most are not, and in fact it has been suggested that only 10 to 15% are.[136] The majority are therefore missing a key ingredient to success, because self-awareness helps us to live and perform better. We are more likely to be happy and healthy, to make sounder decisions, build stronger relationships, perform better at work, communicate more effectively, and gain in confidence, all as a result of enhanced self-awareness.[137] While mental and emotional self-awareness are the principle focus, 'physical' self-awareness helps us to recognise how our bodies are responding to circumstances, and it helps us to take care of ourselves better, recognise stress earlier, and execute healthier behaviours.

From a psychology perspective, it is easiest to divide self-awareness into two components. **Internal** self-awareness means our insight into our thoughts, reactions, and behaviours – our strengths and weaknesses. **External** self-awareness means how much we understand how others see us. Someone might be strong in one, and less strong in the other, as illustrated in table 10.2 (and later in figure 10.2).

| | **High External Self-Awareness** | **Low External Self-Awareness** |
|---|---|---|
| **High Internal Self-Awareness** | You know who you are and how others see you. | You know who you are but don't see what others see. |
| **Low Internal Self-Awareness** | You don't have much understanding of yourself but know how others see you. | You don't have much understanding of yourself nor how others see you. |

**Table 10.2** Self-awareness is a result of our understanding of insights into our own selves (internal self-awareness) and how much we understand how others see us (external self-awareness).

There are many ways to help us to further build a picture of our own self-awareness, and the typical place to start is identifying strengths and weaknesses.

## Strengths, Weaknesses, and the Role of Personality

*Stronger by weakness, wiser men become.*

**Edmund Waller** [iv]

Here we go again, the strengths and weaknesses topic... We have all come across it somewhere, whether it was at school, preparing for our first job interview (who of us hasn't wondered what we 'should' say, rather than being honest?), a programme at work, or an annual appraisal... It all feels a bit like a chore, something we 'have' to do, rather than want to do. But it's worth it; it is part of building self-awareness, it is empowering, and makes life so much easier.

Most people do not have the ability to properly estimate their own strengths and weaknesses without some help. In some there is significant cognitive bias,[v] with people who are very poor at a task tending to grossly overestimate their ability at performing it. This is called the Dunning-Kruger effect, or 'illusory superiority'. Dunning and Kruger studied psychology students, examining their self-assessments of their intellectual skills in logical reasoning, English grammar, and sense of humour.[138] After learning their self-assessment scores, the students were asked to estimate their ranks in the psychology class. The competent students underestimated their class rank, and the incompetent students overestimated theirs. Those who scored in the bottom quartile on tests overestimated their test performance and their abilities. For example, despite test scores that placed a student in the 12th percentile, the participant estimated he or she ranked in the 62nd percentile. This has been confirmed by other studies.[139] Notably though, training in a task can improve people's ability to estimate their own competence at it,[140] and so here we are, back at the subject of the importance of training and deliberate practice.

v. English poet and politician, 1606–1687.

v. This systematic error in thinking occurs when people are processing and interpreting information in the world around them and it affects the decisions and judgments that they make.

## Start with Strengths

'Find your strengths'. 'Build on your strengths'. 'You can only build from your strengths'... These are well-established mantras in human performance programmes. This emphasis on strengths is understandable and has merit, in that we should be able to recognise our strengths and draw positivity from that. Our strengths can be defined in two ways. One way is to focus on strengths that relate to a specific goal. The second way is a more holistic perspective of our overall strengths that influence many of our activities and interactions in life, the bigger picture. The latter is harder to do and takes longer because it is all part of building self-awareness. It takes time – and in fact it is often a continuous process – but the steady investment is usually worth it.

## The Role of Personality

Personality has long been proposed to play a role in dictating our strengths. Initially it was proposed that people can be classified into specific types that reflect who they are and how they will live life. In fact, as long ago as the time of the Roman Empire, the Greek physician, surgeon, and philosopher Galen (~AD 129) proposed the Four Temperaments (sanguine, choleric, melancholic, phlegmatic) as being important descriptors of human beings. It was Carl Jung who, in the early twentieth century, proposed that 'it is one's psychological type which from the outset determines and limits a person's judgment.'[141] In the 1950s the Myers-Briggs Type Indicator (MBTI)[142] became increasingly used as a profiling tool – a test to determine the personality type of individuals as part of job recruitment strategies. The test attempts to assign four categories: introversion or extraversion, sensing or intuition, thinking or feeling, judging or perceiving. It is still in use to this day, and much is written about it; yet it is not validated, is unreliable, and is considered pseudoscience.[143]

The whole subject of categorising people according to a specific 'type' of personality is highly contentious. Instead, it has been proposed that personality *traits* are more appropriate descriptors. These are ingrained behavioural tendencies that are proposed to predict what you will be good at. Psychologists talk about the 'Big Five' traits: Openness,

Conscientiousness, Extraversion, Agreeableness, and Neuroticism (OCEAN). When we focus on performance, these have been proposed to reflect our strengths relating to certain types of jobs, and indeed providing strengths-based performance programmes for the corporate world has become a big industry. Various far more elaborate testing systems, proposing not just five but dozens of traits, are used to define an individual's strengths according to their personality traits. But looking for strengths to identify the right talent to fill a role in a company, and/or to promote employee engagement with a manager, is not the same as establishing ways of achieving a fulfilling performance on a personal level. Furthermore, the premise that personality is the key indicator of our strengths and performance capacity is not proven, and it is a great shame that there is a paucity of published papers in peer-reviewed journals even relating to widely used strengths-based profiling tools. These are commercial products with big followings, but unfortunately without the evidence presented to prove their worth. The popularity of the personality-based approach lies at least partly in the *Barnum (or Forer) effect*.[144] This is the phenomenon that occurs when individuals believe that personality descriptions apply specifically to them (more so than to other people), despite the fact that the description is actually filled with information that applies to everyone. It's a bit like going to the fair, having your fortune read, and it seemingly applies to you but is generic enough that it could apply to many. It is a form of subconscious bias.

So is there any use at all to knowing our traits? Of course there is, because it is part of self-awareness, which is a key component of performance; and our behavioural traits do influence – variably – how we perform in different situations. Moreover, if a strengths-based profiling tool helps to kick-start us reflecting on our strengths and weaknesses, and getting some support as needed, then great. However in truth, the only evidence for a personality trait as a predictor of performance is *conscientiousness*. This trait is the only one of the Six Key Characteristics that is partly inborn and not entirely built through training, but even this can be significantly improved through taking the right steps.

## Embracing Weaknesses

Let's face it, we all have weaknesses, and life would be quite boring if we didn't. Things that we view as weaknesses may not be the things that others see. (For example, many were surprised by Mike Tyson's statement: 'My biggest weakness is my sensitivity. I am too sensitive a person'.) Furthermore, focusing on the weaknesses that matter is key. The famous golfer Jack Nicklaus confessed, 'If I have any weakness, it's probably ice cream... butter pecan', and best-selling author Jackie Collins declared that her weakness was wearing leopard print, but probably those weaknesses didn't stand in the way of their success in life!

We need to be very clear that self-awareness is how we consciously know and understand ourselves: our character, feelings, motives, actions – and yes, our traits. If we are to see ourselves clearly, then we must see not just our strengths, but our weaknesses too. We may be really good at some things, but the other things that we are less good at may be diluting our performance, and addressing them is simply being smart. If a 100-metre sprinter is great in the last 20 metres but terrible out of the blocks, then wouldn't it be a good idea for them to focus on improving their start? Even if it becomes only a bit better, that may be enough to make the difference in the outcome of a race. In the workplace, if an individual's performance in giving a presentation is strengthened by their ability to create great visuals but is then limited by their tendency to rush through them at breakneck speed, isn't it better to work on the latter? These are rather simplistic, specific examples, but other weaknesses can seem more complicated or be more subtle. For example, they may relate to how we react in certain situations or how we interact with people in different environments and in different conditions. Evaluating these areas takes more time and reflection and is part of building self-awareness.

Addressing weaknesses is not an insurmountable task, and in fact, tweaking a weakness can have a much greater impact than trying to 'strengthen a strength'. Deceptively small changes can have seismic impacts, particularly if taken collectively. This is where the commonly used term of 'marginal gains' comes in: making small, incremental improvements in any process, which, when added together, make a significant improvement.

## How to Assess Strengths and Weaknesses

There are no validated systems that make this easy or automated. I have highlighted that there are strengths profiling and other tools that are very popular in the field of self-awareness. They may help to promote a conversation about ourselves and result in some support, which may motivate us to take the whole matter seriously – and bravo if they do. Hopefully the evidence base in peer-reviewed journals to support these tools will appear. However, they do not replace some necessary effort using more simplistic approaches.

For many, the best way of assessing strengths and weaknesses that relate to a specific goal is through the long-used 'Strengths, Weaknesses, Opportunities, Threats' (SWOT) analysis. This tool is as useful as the user makes them; they take time and reflection to do well but can be *very* worthwhile. A SWOT analysis is mostly used with a specific goal in mind, and it is often easier to get some input from others. The individual asks one or more trusted people in their life to assist in identifying their strengths and weaknesses: family, co-workers/mentors, and/or a coach, depending on the circumstances. Opportunities relate to situations and things that they may take advantage of to facilitate their goals, and threats are potential elements that will get in the way.

SWOT analysis is a popular and easy first approach to building self-awareness in relation to a goal, but the process does not end there. Working to build more comprehensive 'whole person' self-awareness should be pursued.

### The Big Picture of Gaining Self-Awareness

The whole process of building self-awareness, enhancing metacognition, and consciously self-monitoring does not happen by accident. It starts with a structured approach to gaining insights, followed by frequent short spells to self-reflect, and being mindful. The Johari Model is a helpful tool in facilitating this.[145] It incorporates four basic elements that are assessed and used as a framework: the Known, Blind, Hidden, and Unknown. Using this model not only relies on self-evaluation but also requires input from others, who must be trusted individuals who know the person, who

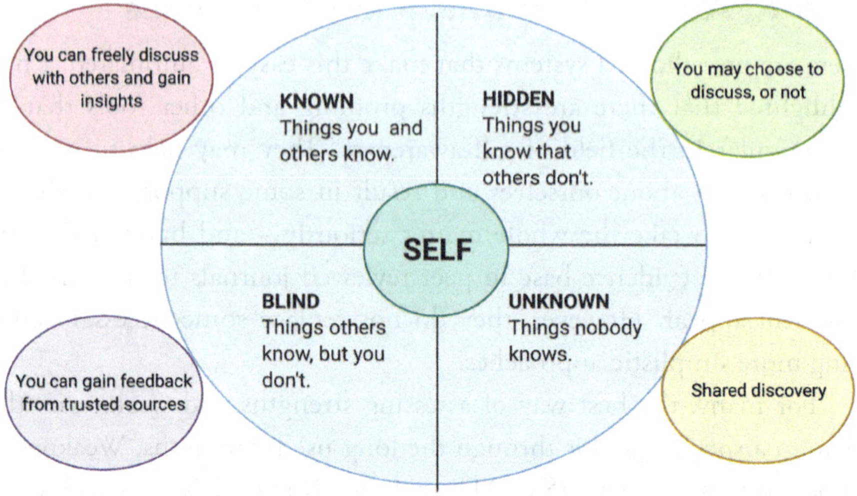


**Figure 10.2** The Johari Window and modelling approaches to enhancing self-awareness.[vi]

are comfortable with expressing their views, and who can add value to any discussion without seeming intimidating or destructive. Typically, people have a tendency to easily highlight strengths of others before they will stray to mentioning weaknesses. Not everyone though!

In the work setting, if a member of a team is not self-aware, that can dilute the efforts of the team. That said, being one of the trusted support team to provide constructive feedback can be very difficult, and only a minority seem comfortable with the approach. That is particularly true for providing feedback to someone more senior, and perhaps this is one reason why those who are in senior positions may become less self-aware: lack of honest feedback.

vi. For a more detailed description of the Johari Window, go to https://en.wikipedia.org/wiki/Johari_window.

In this model, the individual (let's say, you) chooses from a wide selection of adjectives (provided in the process) that you think apply to yourself. Your trusted others do the same, selecting those that they think apply to you.

- Those that both you and others agree on go into the KNOWN category.
- Those that you think apply to you but the others don't, go into the HIDDEN category.
- Things that others think apply, but you don't, go into the BLIND category.
- All the other adjectives that no one has chosen go into the UNKNOWN category.
- This template then forms the starting point for conversations and reflection on your strengths and weaknesses.

## Time to Reflect

Once insights are gained, through whatever means, regular self-reflection follows. We are so often told, 'Take time to reflect', but when someone says that to us, we often grumble, 'Time?! Who has time to spare?!' But just fifteen minutes of reflection – at the end of the day to consider what was good and less good, or before the day when we might consider what lies ahead – are found to lead to better performance and happiness and less burn-out.[146] Using this time to reflect on our thoughts, emotions, and behaviours in relation to specific events assists with the ongoing development of self-awareness. Experiences we have strongly influence those reflections and can add significant benefits. These planned regular short periods dedicated to self-reflection are enough to start to build the foundations, and these can be incorporated into general mindfulness activities that are performed more regularly through the day. Mindfulness is described in the next chapter, Vitality.

*The worst of all deceptions is self-deception.*

**Plato**

## Key Messages:

- Self-awareness means recognising our thoughts, emotions, and behaviours. It means recognising how our bodies and minds work, and how we respond to challenges, circumstances, and our environment.
- Self-awareness is a fundamental step to enhancing human performance in many ways that are evident in day-to-day life.
- Whether we like it or not, understanding not just our strengths, but also our weaknesses is part of learning to perform well in different ways.
- Focusing on weaknesses as well as strengths is healthy and positive and is essential to gain self-awareness.
- Identifying some areas to focus on for improvement – be it related to small goals or the big picture of life – is the starting point.
- There are no easy, reliable shortcuts, and commercial tools may help but will only get the user so far.
- Individual empowerment is key.
- Having the support of trusted others, and planning time for dedicated reflection, are all part of the process of enhancing self-awareness.

# 11

# Vitality

*It is health that is the real wealth, and not pieces of gold and silver*

**Mahatma Gandhi**

## What Health Is Really About: Vitality

*Health and well-being*... what does that actually mean? The World Health Organization says that health is 'a state of complete physical, mental and social well-being and not merely the absence of disease or infirmity'.[147] So 'well-being' is inherent to health and we don't actually need to state it as a separate commodity, but we do so, probably to emphasise the importance of a sense of happiness or satisfaction with life. When it comes to performance, health and well-being are extremely important, but we need to reach beyond that to get the most from ourselves. That means placing added emphasis on energy, drive, and positivity.

Positivity has already been highlighted earlier in the discussion about self-effectiveness, the power of self-belief. It has a big impact on our health and on how we perform. Positive thinking is linked to living longer, better heart health, lower rates of depression, greater resistance to the common cold, greater psychological and physical well-being, and better coping skills. How positivity results in all of these benefits isn't clear, although it is considered to be at least in part due to lower levels of inflammation in our bodies due to managing stress better. Also, people who are positive thinkers are also more likely to have healthier lifestyles. A focus on positivity acts as a kick-starter to any nutrition, fitness, or other health programme and then continues as an ongoing priority; it will make any performance journey far more enjoyable and more likely to lead to a successful outcome. On the flip side, negative thinking makes it a lot more likely we will fail, and this is the most common reason for failure to succeed in a health/fitness-related goal. We start well, encounter a setback or do not see the rate of progress we expected, and negative thinking kicks in... Many people who have tried and failed several times on a new health regime then fall into the trap of starting out *expecting* the plan to fail.

*Whether you think you can, or you think you can't—you're right.*

**Henry Ford**

It is positivity that transforms health and well-being into aliveness, and it is that same positivity that helps to translate aliveness into performance. It follows that no matter how much we focus on the importance of fitness, nutrition, sleep, and tactics to make things fall into place more easily, the positivity of thinking and actions and the energy it creates is the critical thing. This aliveness, this positivity, blends with our health and well-being – and that end product is vitality. Vitality is *pivotal* to achieving fulfilling performances.

*Vitality! That's the pursuit of life, isn't it?*

**Katharine Hepburn**

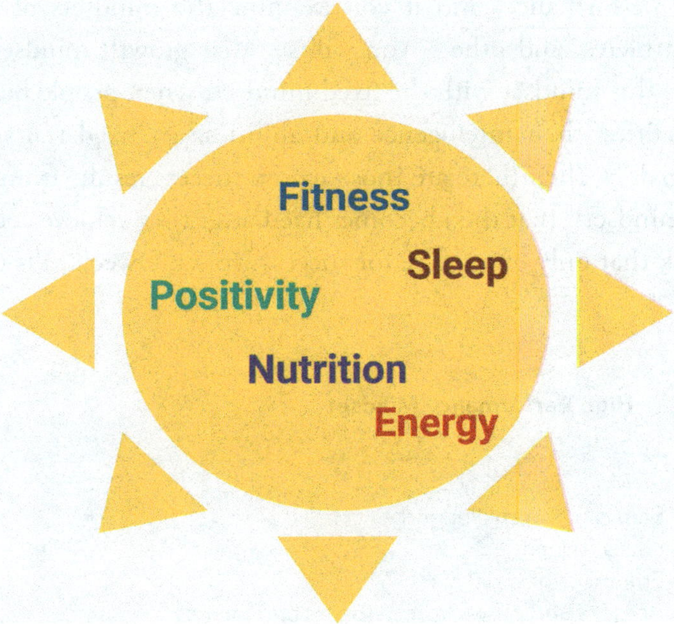


**Figure 11.1** Components of Vitality.

## Positivity and the Performance Mindset

The positivity that is part of vitality is what underpins the ***performance mindset***, reflecting a positive way of thinking about things, a set of attitudes that influence our decision making and approach, a set of beliefs that reflect how we see ourselves, our intelligence, our talents, and our capabilities. Mindset often reflects personal identity and beliefs, and it acts as a powerful influence over choices and behaviours. No doubt it will be apparent by now how strongly this overlaps with self-efficacy.

Having the right mindset is essential to performing consistently well: those who do not think like a high performer cannot act like one. A positive mindset allows the freedom to explore new things, to create new beliefs, to learn and thrive. The American psychologist Carol Dweck describes this as a 'growth mindset';[148] but perhaps considering it as a 'learn, stretch, and thrive mindset' is a better descriptor. It is the ability to enjoy being challenged by new things, to stretch our thinking and beliefs to learn, to accept and respond positively to setbacks and failures, and to thrive as a result. Whatever you want to call it, it is the basis for high performance, and if you examine the mindsets of successful leaders, athletes, and others, you will see that growth mindsets prevail. Compare this mindset with the fixed mindset, when people believe their basic qualities, their intelligence and abilities, are fixed traits and can't be changed.[149] Then there are those whose success results from an initial growth mindset[vii] that then becomes fixed after they achieve certain goals and think that only one recipe for success works. Dweck calls this 'CEO disease'.[150]

| The High Performance Mindset |
| --- |
| • Self-belief<br>• Enjoys being challenged<br>• Loves to learn<br>• Embraces new beliefs<br>• Accepts and grows from setbacks and failures<br>• Is willing to make the effort<br>• Has a clear structure and plan<br>• Gets support when needed |

**Table 11.1** Characteristics of those with a high performance mindset.

## The Power of Positive Thinking: Facing Pressure and Managing Stress

In any discussion about performance, the concept of stress and pressure will inevitably crop up. They are two words used interchangeably in relation to dealing with day-to-day challenges, and both are highly relevant to performing, but they mean different things. Understanding stress responses, the meaning of pressure, and how to channel both positively is key to greater well-being and better performance.

***Stress*** is a word widely used and abused. Its best definition is that it is *the body's physiological, emotional, and mental reactions to feeling*

vii. To test your own mindset, take the online quiz at: Lewis Swift, 'Interactive Quiz: Fixed vs. Growth Mindsets', London Academy of IT, 10 February 2015, https://www.londonacademyofit.co.uk/blog/interactive-quiz-fixed-vs-growth-mindset.

*threatened, triggered by one or more stressors in our environment.* The **acute** stress response is an evolutionary function, a complex phenomenon involving multiple systems in the body that are primed to respond for good reason: *survival.* These responses allow us to deal with threats, but it is when our stress responses are inappropriate or prolonged (**chronic**) that stress moves from being an essential biological entity to having negative implications that harm our health, well-being, and performance.

***Pressure*** is different from stress. Pressure relates to our responses to an expectation, often self-imposed, to perform well in a situation. Feeling under pressure can trigger positive or negative responses, that determine how we behave and ultimately how we perform.

## Acute Stress Responses: What Happens?

The term *stress* was first used in the 1930s by hormone specialist Hans Selye,[151] who noted that, after exposing animals to various noxious stimuli, they all showed a similar reaction that he called 'General Adaptation Syndrome (GAS)'. He described three phases:

1 an *alarm phase* in which an organism identifies a stressor or a threat and the body mounts an alarm response, then

2 a *resistance phase* in which the body attempts to adapt and cope with the stressor, and lastly

3 an *exhaustion phase* in which the resources are eventually depleted in the face of sustained stress and the body is unable to maintain normal function.

The alarm phase is mostly what we now call the 'acute stress response', whereas the other two phases represent chronic stress.

Acute stress responses are the easiest to understand from a biological 'survival' perspective. The perception of danger sets off an automatic response system, known as the '*fight-or-flight*' response, which prepares an animal to meet a threat or to flee from it. A simple example is a car driving towards us at speed when we are crossing the road – we see the threat and 'automatically' jump out the way. Another example is when a colleague gets aggressive with us in a meeting. We can't jump out the

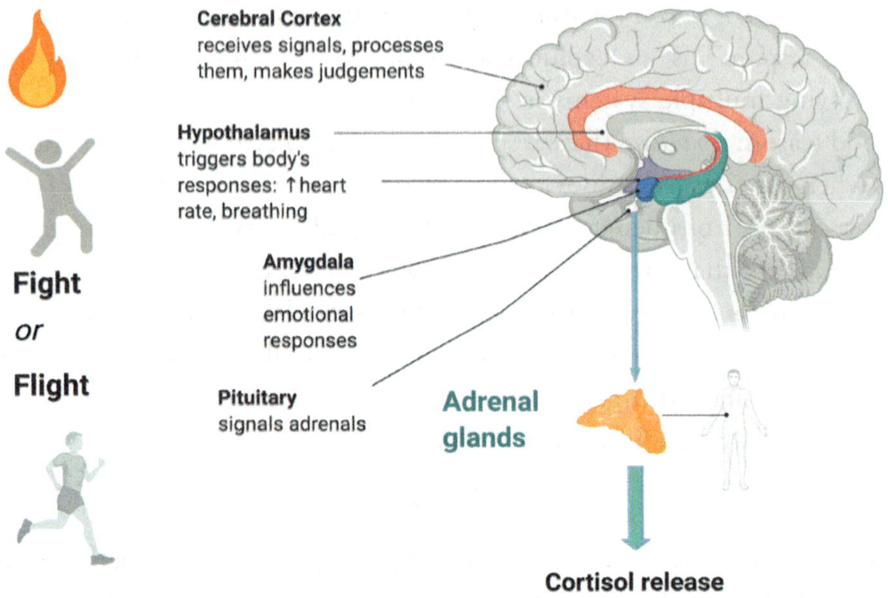


**Figure 11.2** The acute stress response.

way physically, but we may become aware of some of the physiological mechanisms that are associated with stress. For example, our heart rate rises, our mouth feels dry, we may notice a sense of anxiety, restlessness, or fear.

What actually happens in the background when we are exposed to acute stressors? Firstly, the thinking bit of the brain (cortex) identifies a situation. Then the emotional bit of the brain (amygdala) identifies it as a danger. Another bit of the brain, the hypothalamus, then organises the response to the threat by sending a signal to the pituitary gland, which sends another signal to the adrenal glands (near the kidneys), and adrenaline, noradrenaline, and cortisol are released. These are the stress hormones.

Cortisol is a simple steroid hormone, and it is very, very powerful. It is essential for life, and just like other physiological processes in the body, it has a 'circadian rhythm'[viii] with higher levels in the morning and

viii. A circadian rhythm is a biological internal process that regulates the sleep-wake cycle and repeats approximately every twenty-four hours. See the further discussion in chapter 17, 'Sleep to Succeed'.

lower levels at night in healthy individuals (the opposite to the sleep hormone melatonin). It can significantly affect the hippocampus in the temporal lobe in the brain that regulates motivation, emotion, learning, and memory.

When cortisol is released, it raises alertness and helps us to stay motivated and focused on the task at hand. It stimulates the release of sugar into the blood from organs like the liver and kidneys, and fat is released from storage sites, so there is plenty of energy available to deal with the stressor. Cortisol also increases heart rate and blood pressure so that blood is pumped to working muscles. Breathing rate increases, which with the increased circulation allows more oxygen to be distributed to vital areas. The senses, including sight and hearing, become sharper. This is all to prepare for the 'flight' response in the acute situation, but it also reduces brain metabolism, immune responses, and growth and repair of tissues as the body systems focus on dealing with threat.

The threat is recognised and responded to, even before the brain has had time to consciously process what is happening. When the threat subsides, the stress response is dampened down by other processes driven by the parasympathetic nervous system, which is the 'rest and digest' nervous system as opposed to the 'fight or flight' sympathetic nervous system. Heart rate and breathing settle, blood pressure reverts to normal, and the stress hormones are no longer released. This can take minutes to hours.

Most people assume that feeling acute stress is always a bad sign, but it is not; it is an inbuilt survival mechanism. Nevertheless, there are certainly some significant situations in life that undoubtedly impose negative stress. The most frequent cause of acute negative stress is *overload*, where the demands on us outweigh our energy and internal resources to deal with those demands effectively, or at least we perceive that they do, and we feel out of control. It is clear that there is a wide inter-individual variation in stress responses, and while the reasons are not fully understood, it is also clear that those responses can be modified through training. Elevated stress levels can impede focus and attention and can impair working memory, retrieval of information from memory, and decision making. These are just a few mechanisms by which acute

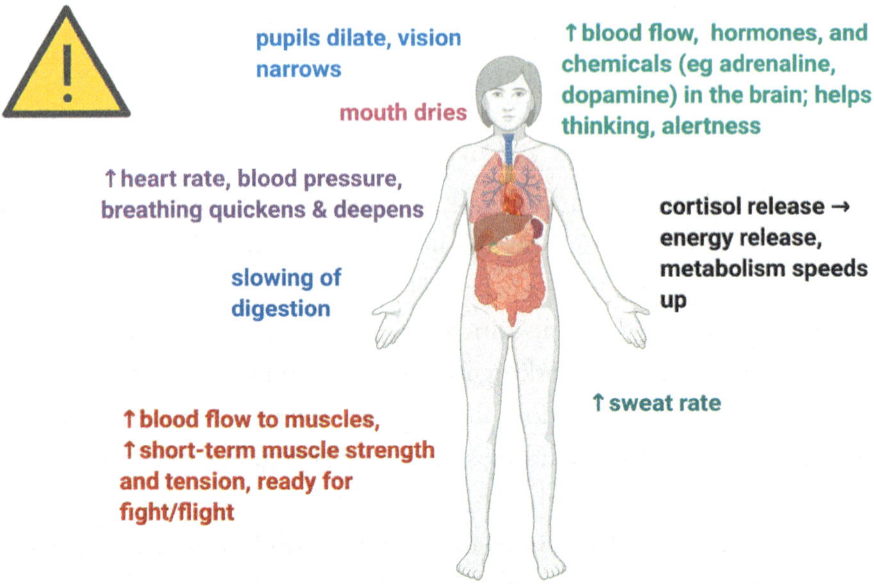


**Figure 11.3** The principal physiological changes in the body when exposed to acute stress.

stress can have negative impacts on performance. These effects appear to be determined by the individual's appraisal of the demands and resources of a situation, the relationship between the stressor and the task, and factors such as coping styles, locus of control, and social supports.[152] Hence, part of preventing the detrimental effects of acute stress lies in perception of stress, its implications, and individual strategies for coping.

The fundamental effects of stress on the brain have been demonstrated using fMRI studies, which found that those who are more susceptible to stress show differences in brain activity in the process, particularly in the prefrontal cortex, the executive control headquarters. This indicates that cognition and executive control are potentially affected by stress in those who have the greatest stress response.[153]

It is important to note that in many performance situations, stress can work in a positive way ('eustress'), assisting with readiness for a situation/event. Those who learn to use stress well can truly thrive on challenges and perform well as a result. In most performance situations it is a matter of perception, such as whether the individual sees something as a threat or as a challenge.

## Chronic Stress

We all have episodes of acute stress. If our strategies and coping mechanisms kick in well, no harm should occur, and indeed it may serve a purpose (typically that's when there is eustress). However, when stress becomes chronic, that's a whole new ballgame, and a very negative one at that. Prolonged stress responses occur when there is one or more persisting perceived 'threats' or hassles in life that result in ongoing adverse physiological and psychological events.

In chronic stress, sustained cortisol levels result in sugar being released into the blood stream that increases the risk of obesity and diabetes. Heart rate and blood pressure rise, the risk of heart disease goes up, there is damage to memory and cognition, mood swings and often depression can occur, and it becomes increasingly difficult to focus on tasks. Fatigue is a very common outcome of chronic stress, and often the most notable feature. It makes people underperform, and their health and well-being slide downhill.

Stress is 'pro-inflammatory', meaning that it drives inflammation, is damaging to tissues, and wreaks havoc with the immune system, whose function it is to protect from infections and a range of other illnesses including cancers. The reproductive system is also affected: in men testosterone levels and sperm counts can fall, in women menstrual irregularities and worsened PMT occur, and in all, libido can often be affected. Unpleasant gastrointestinal effects also are common with heartburn, reflux, and poor absorption of foods. Muscles become tense and painful, and headaches are common.

Then there are the effects of stress on sleep, and when sleep is affected there are further knock-on effects on health, including greater risks of developing diseases and negative impacts on mood and cognition. (This will be discussed in chapter 17.) Daily habits are also affected; stress can cause overeating and other poor eating behaviours, which in turn are harmful and can perpetuate the stress process.

Eventually, there is *burnout:* extreme exhaustion, lack of well-being, inability to cope, reduced performance, and major health issues. Experts disagree on the exact definition, and there is no easy way to measure it, but most understand the term. Mood often drops, and burnout can be confused with depression. Prevention by early recognition of stress and early intervention is key.

## Dealing with Stress: Reframing Thinking and Mindfulness

Reframing our thinking towards a positive mindset creates more positive behaviours and better results.[ix] This, of course, is not easy. For some people it can be the area that needs a lot of work. We all have some negative thoughts, and knowing what to do with them is the challenge. There is an aboriginal tradition designed to remove peoples' troubles, where the community members link hands with the troubled person at one end of the chain and with a large tree at the other end. The person with the troubles symbolically passes it to the next person, who passes it to the next, and on until the final person passes the trouble to the tree. This is known as 'Treeing' or parking negative thoughts or feelings and

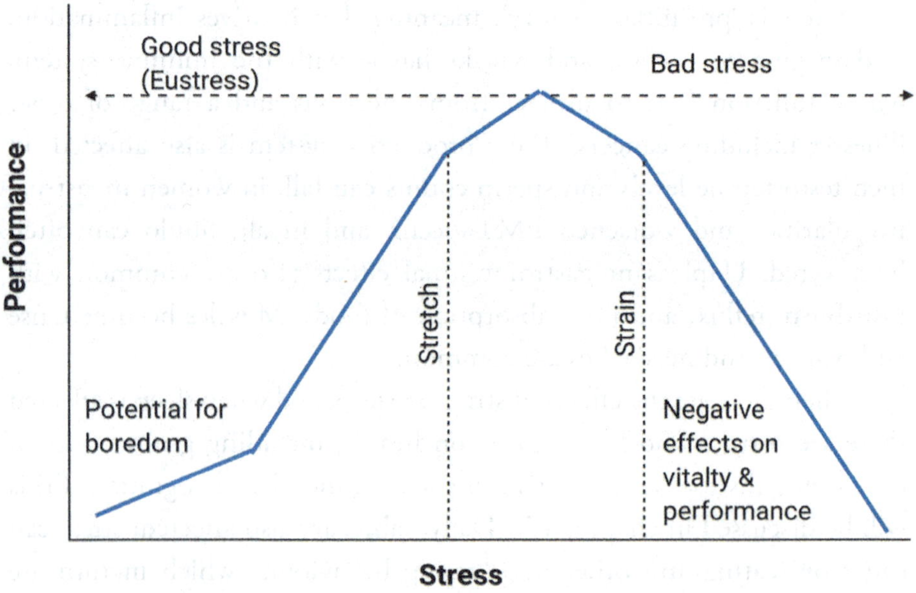


**Figure 11.4** The human function curve: Some stress has positive effects on performance, but getting the balance right is key.

ix. This is the basis for cognitive behavioural therapy.

having a systematic way of doing this. For example, a mental box where we put the thoughts, or writing them down and putting the page away in a drawer and refocusing on the positive. Whatever works.

*For there is nothing either good or bad, but thinking makes it so.*

**Hamlet, act 2 scene 2**

## Mindfulness

Mindfulness is conscious awareness of the moment and our responses to it. It is about 'knowing what is going on inside and outside ourselves, moment by moment'.[154] It enables us to connect with our bodies and our minds and recognise our responses, including signs of early stress. It enhances our awareness of our thoughts and emotions such that we can untangle what may seem complex issues, see solutions more clearly, and channel our responses positively. Mindfulness focuses on the present moment; it is analytical in a way, such that we observe how we are thinking and feeling about a situation and our environment. It is conscious awareness, noticing elements that often escape our attention. It is not just sitting there doing nothing in silence!

Mindfulness and its potential benefits have received much interest in recent times, as evidenced by the number of related publications increasing six-fold in the past ten years. Many of these contain no true science, but there is evidence that mindfulness has beneficial effects on health in general: improvements in mental health,[155] immunity,[156] and reduced pain levels,[157] with reports that it has the same effects as exercise and drugs on mood and well-being.[158] In the workplace, research shows that mindfulness training reduces emotional exhaustion/burnout, stress, psychological distress, depression, and anxiety, and improves sleep, relaxation, self-compassion, and a sense of personal accomplishment.[159]

A study from Harvard Medical School examined the effects of mindfulness training on stress and well-being, using fMRI to examine changes in the brain.[160] They recruited people who had never meditated before and divided them into two groups: one group had an eight-week mindfulness meditation intervention (Mindfulness Based Stress

Reduction, MBSR), and the other control group did not. The eight-week training group had a weekly meditation class and a recommended forty minutes a day of meditation, while the control group did not go through the mindfulness classes or meditate at all. Before and after the eight weeks, the volume of grey matter in the brains of the subjects was analysed using fMRI. The results showed that the brains of the control group had not changed, but the brains of those who had trained and practiced mindfulness had increased in four different areas: (1) the area associated with focus and self-relevance, (2) the area concerned with learning and memory, (3) the area for perspective taking, empathy and compassion, and (4) the area that aids in sleep, amongst other things. Also, there was a decrease in the volume of the amygdala, which is the area associated with fear and perceived stress.

Equally importantly, the changes in brain structure with meditation were correlated with reductions in stress, anxiety, mind-wandering, and insomnia, as well as increased quality of life as compared to those who did not practice meditation. The researchers also measured cortisol, a stress hormone, and found decreased levels of cortisol within the participants who underwent mindfulness meditation intervention.

Practicing and performing mindfulness can take different forms, from formal meditation to more informal exercises such as focusing on experiencing a single moment. They vary in delivery mode, from one-on-one training, to online work, or even self-taught through some reading. Many programmes are based on the Mindfulness Based Stress Reduction training, as mentioned earlier, developed by Kabat-Zinn,[161] which was originally developed to treat chronic pain. It is an intensive programme, consisting of eight 2.5-hour weekly sessions and one 7-hour day of silence, with 45 minutes of daily exercise at home, 6 days per week with supportive CDs and set tasks. It includes body scan (paying attention to what the body is feeling), sitting meditation, simple movement exercises such as walking, yoga exercises, while paying attention to what the body is feeling, informal meditation activities, focusing on the moment. You can see how this also relates to **self-awareness**. Many do not have the time to invest in such programmes, but simpler, shorter training, even fifteen minutes per day, with or without a coach, can be highly beneficial.

It is the regularity of the training that is key – yet again, it is all about regular, deliberate practice.

The key is to incorporate mindfulness across all activities of our lives. It enhances relationships, mental clarity, confidence, decision making, creativity, and well-being. Mindfulness is for everyone, not just those with health issues; there is good evidence that it makes lives better and helps people to perform. Mindfulness can be incorporated across all elements of vitality and performance: how we eat, sleep, plan, exercise, relax, and interact.

## Preventing Burnout

Understanding stress, recognizing how it affects us, identifying warning signs of persisting stress, and having strategies to deal with it will enhance well-being, health, and performance. Identifying stressors – the predictable ones – is an essential exercise in all of this and allows us to prepare for specific scenarios to use when practicing techniques to minimise their effects, and channel them to the good.

There are a few key elements to preventing burnout due to chronic stress. Firstly, understand it. Secondly, recognise the signals when it happens (self-awareness, mindfulness). Thirdly, take measures to counteract it and to make it less likely we will be affected by it in the first place. That is achieved through self-effectiveness, optimising components of vitality, and mindfulness.

For some groups, such as employers, coaches, and clinicians, being able to measure stress helps to develop targeted intervention strategies. Some find it useful on an individual basis too, although for many, constantly measuring stress may in itself be stressful! For many, introducing more mindfulness and awareness of how they respond to and manage stressors will be more productive. Just acknowledging 'I am beginning to feel stressed' can be enough to trigger adaptive responses. Being able to identify one's physiological responses to stress can help us to tune in to the warning signs without needing anything more sophisticated to measure it.

For those who *do* feel monitoring stress objectively will help, there are a few approaches. Stress scores like the Perceived Stress Score[162] are more research tools than day-to-day methods, but completing a score every few weeks will help to highlight stress status and can prompt insights.

**Technologies** are now also widely promoted; some may be helpful and undoubtedly there will be further positive developments in this respect. Elevated resting heart rate (RHR) is one sign of stress, illness, or poor recovery from activities the day before. You can check your pulse yourself, when fully rested such as on waking in the morning. However, the best measure is probably the night-time resting heart rate, and the best way to assess RHR in general is to wear a device like a wrist band, ring, or even a smartwatch. Once we know what your resting heart rate is, if it goes up by >5 beats/minute it is a sign we are one or more of the following: stressed, not recovered from the day before/overtraining, dehydrated, sleep deprived, or ill. Note that some medications also influence our heart rates.

Other markers may be useful, for example electrodermal activity (EDA), also known as skin conductance response (SCR), which reflects change in sweat level, are measured by some devices, but their reliability is quite varied.

Smartwatches, wrist bands, and other monitoring systems also offer 'stress scores'. The methods by which these are calculated is not transparent; another example of the black boxes.

*Heart rate variability* (HRV) is used by many tech companies to measure stress. Simply put, it is the time interval between heartbeats. Our hearts don't beat like metronomes; there is variation depending on the demands on us, our health, and our fitness status. This variability is regulated by the autonomic nervous system, composed of the sympathetic and parasympathetic systems. Remember these? They are the systems that trigger the 'fight or flight' response (sympathetic) or the 'rest and digest' (parasympathetic). We need both to survive and thrive, and HRV indicates how well both systems are working. In *general,* a high HRV is good and a low HRV is not so good. This makes sense if we consider that a higher HRV means that your autonomic nervous system is versatile in responding to demands imposed on you, and this is reflected in variation in the interval between heartbeats. It would be nice to think that we just need to measure HRV and know it represents one thing, like stress. But unfortunately, it's not that straight forward. HRV is actually a highly complex measurement that can be influenced by a range of other factors, such as hormones, metabolism, breathing, and our state of health. Genetics play a significant role (as they do with most things), meaning there is significant inter-individual variation. It is how the HRV changes from day to day in an individual that matters. So, although HRV is a relevant physiological measure, it isn't just measuring one thing. It is measuring our overall ANS (automatic nervous system) status, which can reflect our general health, recovery, and stress levels as a whole. That's still highly relevant as long as its meaning is understood. The real concern about using this as a 'stress and recovery' marker is the method of measurement and the reliability of devices to measure what they say they do. Measures can be inaccurate if not taken under the right conditions, and different technologies use different approaches to measurement and calculation of HRV, some of which are far from valid. Some also blend HRV measurements with other measures and express the result as a number reflecting recovery, stress, strain, and others – but again without presenting any evidence as to their validity. There may be some good devices out there, but there are many bad ones. Again - beware black boxes.

## What's the Difference between Stress and Pressure?

*Man is not troubled by events, but by how he interprets them.*

**Epictetus**

Feeling under pressure is often self-imposed because we want a successful outcome to a task: a presentation to our boss, serving an ace to win the match on the tennis court, giving a recital. In pressure situations the psychological and physiological reactions that occur can help or hinder success. When it is a hindrance, the fear of potential embarrassment and failure disrupts performance through triggering uncontrolled stress responses; we stop thinking clearly, and the skills and behaviours we may have practiced carefully start to fall apart. We start to self-doubt, and over-think things, such that basic skills we would often perform automatically and subconsciously (i.e., habits) start to come into conscious thinking, and performance deteriorates. That's what is described as 'choking' in a sports setting, and the word applies to most other performance settings too. When performers are 'in the zone' they will draw on their subconscious, their habits, to perform well. Often, if asked after the event what they were thinking at the time, they will usually say 'not much'; they just felt fully in the moment and in sync with the process. Psychologists also call this the ***Flow State***[163] – i.e., being fully immersed in the process, fully focused and in control, energised, and enjoying the activity. It is a term frequently used in human performance literature. Achieving a flow state cannot be forced, but there are some essential components to achieve it.

| |
|---|
| **Preparation** |
| **Practice** |
| **Ability to focus** |
| **Confidence** |
| **Self-respect** |

**Table 11.2** Necessary requirements to achieve a flow state.

Pressure will often start well in advance of a scheduled event. Distorted thinking can contribute; magnification of the importance of something and the consequences of failure will often create a perception of threat and trigger stress responses inappropriately. ***Cognitive appraisal*** helps us to prevent this. This is the process by which we assess situations, examine whether we have the abilities to deal with it, and interpret whether we see the situation as a challenge or a threat. Essentially it means *stop and reflect*. This is an important part of planning and preparation; it will often help someone to see the big picture and plan how they can deal with it. What are the true consequences of not succeeding? Is it really as catastrophic as they think? Most situations that feel 'pressured' are not 'once in a lifetime' opportunities. Additionally, how do they define a successful outcome? Does their performance have to be perfect? The answer has got to be *No.*

Most people will have had experiences of unsuccessful outcomes in pressure situations and think 'I don't know why I did that', when their thinking and behaviours have gone AWOL during the situation, often in spite of thinking they were prepared for it. But the trick is to reflect on these experiences and consider how they might have done things differently – this is all part of the learning process. *Every experience at least serves a purpose, even if the outcome was not good.* What is important is that negative experiences and a fear of failure should not lead to aversion behaviours: avoidance of taking on challenges to avoid the possibility of making a mistake. This is a big barrier to progress, and part of cognitive appraisal involves reflecting on whether the consequences of failure really are so significant that we shouldn't try to take an opportunity. '*If you aren't in it, you can't win it.*'

## Rising to the Challenge: The Skills of Dealing with Stress and Pressure in the Context of Performance

We can work to reduce stresses in our lives; that's smart. But we can't avoid all stress, and part of developing as a high performer is encountering new stresses and learning how to deal with them, without allowing them to exert undue pressure on us that adversely affects our performance. If we consider some of the pressured and potentially stressful situations that many people deal with on a daily basis, it is easy to see that it is possible to become skilled at dealing with stress in a positive way. Firemen in a blaze, a paramedic at a road accident, a doctor doing a complex operation, a pro basketball player on the free throw line to win the game, a trader on a volatile day on the markets... Most observers would perceive the challenges those people face as full of pressure and stressful. The point is, those people typically will say they thrive on these situations; that's why they do what they do, and it's not by luck. They do not perceive the situations as negative pressure. While perception of stress is partly 'wired' genetically and from experiences in our early development, performing under pressure is optimised through training, experience, and purposeful practice that allows confidence to build and perceptions of challenges to adapt in a positive way. It is the perception that something is a threat, combined with a fear of failure, that leads to adverse stress responses. Most high performers will say they need to feel some stress to perform best, and they consider 'pressure' in a positive sense. Sensing the heart rate has increased, feeling those butterflies in the stomach – high performers recognise the signs and know it's time to step up with confidence. They take control, recognise it, and channel it.

## What's Next...

Before we move onto the other elements relating to vitality – exercise, nutrition and sleep – it is timely to gain insights into a central element that influences these elements of health and well-being: **chronobiology.**

### Key Messages:

- When it comes to performance, health and well-being are extremely important, but we need to reach beyond that to get the most from ourselves. That means placing added emphasis on energy, drive, and positivity.
- The performance mindset is one of growth and learning.
- Acute stress is a survival mechanism that involves physiological responses.
- Self-awareness and mindfulness help us to recognise acute stress and to channel it such that it can serve a positive purpose, or at least be controlled.
- Chronic stress is harmful to health, well-being and performance. Prevention is key.
- Stress and pressure are not the same.
- Pressure is largely due to expectations, often self-imposed.
- Achieving a flow state helps pressure to be channelled positively.

# 12

# Chronobiology

## Timing Is Everything

*Observe due measure, for right timing is in all things the most important factor.*

**Hesiod, Greek didactic poet (~800 BC)**

*Timing is everything.* We hear it all the time, and clearly from the above quote, it is not a new concept. What does this really mean in relation to performance? Simply put, timing can make things easy when otherwise they are not, and it can mean the difference between success and failure. Timing doesn't just involve 'peaking' at the right time for an event. It relates to the way we schedule the more routine things in life, to optimise how effective we may be, to make the effort worthwhile, to make it all work. Timing of what we do and when is important partly because of our '**chronobiology**' (literally 'time biology'), which involves our internal ('biological') clocks, our circadian rhythms, and our chronotype (the times of day we function best at certain things).

Our bodies are full of internal clocks that keep everything working. These little clocks are governed by a master clock in our brain that acts like an orchestra conductor, controlling all of the other clocks, which collectively regulate the rhythms of our bodies. These rhythms are called **circadian rhythms** – daily cycles that have huge effects on how our bodies function; they are critical to health.

Circadian rhythms can influence sleep-wake cycles, hormone release, eating habits and digestion, body temperature, and other important bodily functions as well as our mood, cognition, and alertness. Alertness, cognitive performance, memory, body temperature, and blood pressure are at their highest during daytime (awake). In contrast, secretion of the hormone melatonin, muscle relaxation, and sleep pressure are at their highest during the night (sleep). In most sporting activities, our circadian rhythms are optimal for performance in the early evening, when reaction

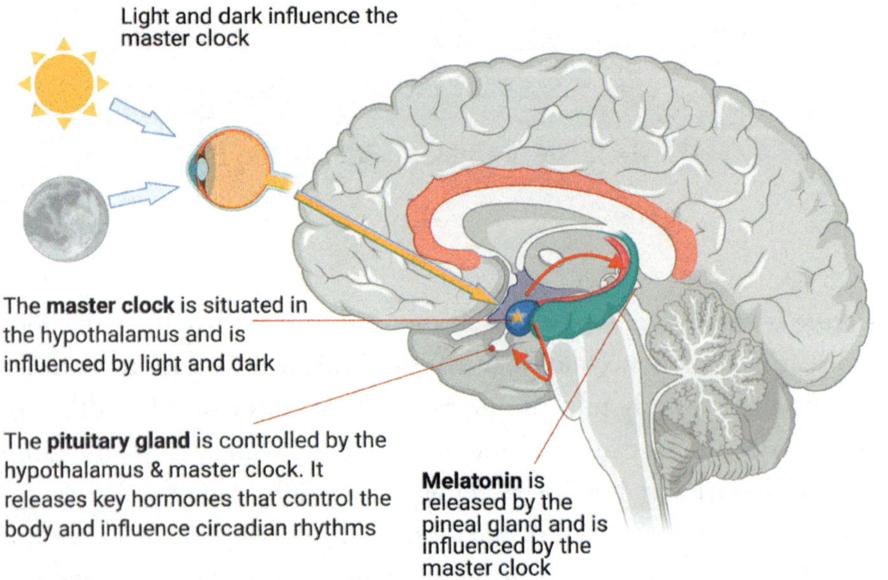


**Figure 12.1** The master clock influences different parts of the brain.

time to light and sound is the fastest; the evening is the time of day when the majority of world records have been broken. Interestingly, activities that require fine motor control and accuracy, such as hand steadiness and balance, are best in the morning.[164]

Biological clocks that run fast or slow can result in disrupted or 'desynchronised' circadian rhythms. These have been linked to various chronic health conditions, such as sleep disorders, obesity, diabetes, depression, bipolar disorder, and seasonal affective disorder.

## Clocks, Cycles, and Chronotypes

Our circadian rhythms mean that for most functions, we follow a cycle of peak, dip, and recovery, the timings of which are largely influenced by our internal clocks. These clocks are partly genetically programmed, but lots of other factors can influence them, for better or for worse. Although our internal clocks' settings are quite individual, people generally can be divided into three types, which are called '**chronotypes**' (literally, 'time types'), also called 'circadian typology'. These three types are morningness (**Lark**), eveningness (**Owl**), and intermediate (**Third Bird**). Statistics vary, but it is said that about 20% of the adult population are Larks, 20% are Owls, and 60% are Third Birds.

Although our chronotype is partly genetically set, it is different between genders, it can change with age, and it is affected by environmental light.[165] When we are children, up until around the age of eight, we are most likely Larks.[166] Then things shift dramatically, such that by early/mid-teens we are Owls. Then in late adolescence/early adulthood we change to our largely genetically set type. Importantly, while chronotype says much about an individual's peak functioning times, it does not specify a personality type, in spite of some claims that it does.

### Establishing Chronotypes

There are various methods used to evaluate an individual's chronotype.[x] However, it is also easy to identify one's type through a simple calculation:

x. An example of chronotype evaluation can be found at the Worldwide Experimental Platform, 'MCTQ', https://www.thewep.org/documentations/mctq.

On non-work days establish what time you go to sleep and what time you wake up, then calculate the mid-point of sleep.

- If it is before 03:30, then you are a Lark.
- If it is after 05:30, then you are an Owl.
- If it is between 03:30 and 05:30, then you are a Third Bird.

## Why Is Chronotype Important?

As you will probably have sensed at this stage, our chronotype largely influences how we perform at different times of the day, whether that relates to our mental arousal (alertness, vigilance, and analytical thinking), our creativity, our physical function, or performing other tasks. Larks tend to be at their peak mental arousal early to midmorning, meaning they should perform their most difficult tasks, those that require greatest alertness and analytical thinking, at that time. Owls are at peak mental arousal in the later afternoon or evening, and Third Birds peak somewhere around late morning. The best time for tasks that involve more creative thinking may for some be when mental arousal levels are lower. For example, Larks and Third Birds are often more creative in the evening.[167] The typical recommendations for Larks and Third Birds to time what to do and when is shown in figure 12.2. The timings shown contrast to those for Owls, who are generally better at cognitive tasks in the later afternoon/evening and are more creative late morning.

Of course, chronobiology applies to everyone, and many activities we perform involve interacting with others. Understanding the chronotypes of co-workers in teams helps to schedule interactions accordingly, which should enhance individual and team performances. In particular, identifying the Owls amongst the team allows scheduling of meetings with Owl type colleagues late in the day.

Being an Owl can be more challenging than being one of the other types. Since most people are either Larks or Third Birds, their preferences for scheduling will not suit the Owls. Learning how to work around this is important for the Owls in order to optimise their performance. For example, when Owls have early-morning meetings, they many need to prepare down to the last detail the night before. Knowing our chronotype

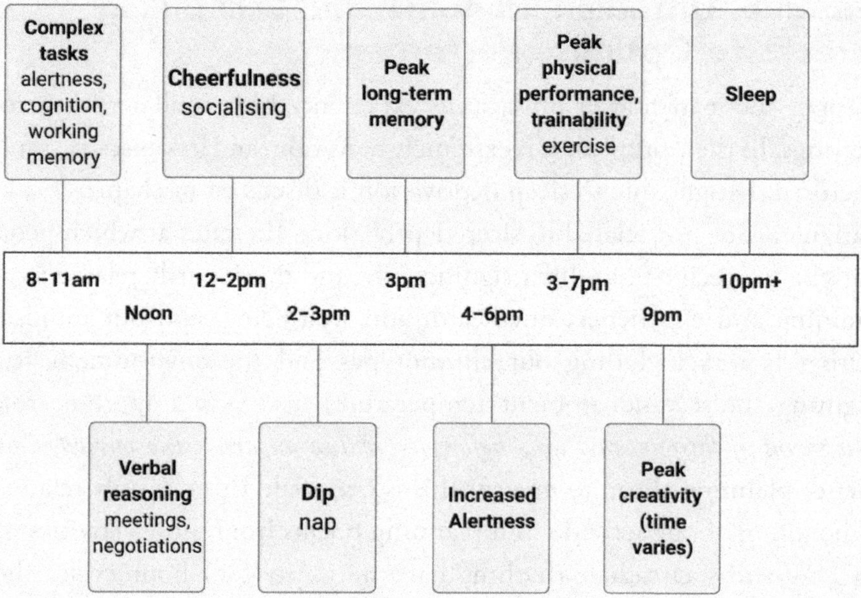


**Figure 12.2** The best times of the day for Larks and Third Birds to perform specific things, based on chronobiology. (Owls typically peak in cognitive tasks in the latter part of the day and are more creative late morning.)

and using this knowledge to influence our planning and sleep schedule is discussed in chapter 17, 'Sleep to Succeed', when the influence of circadian rhythms on our performance is also further detailed. Owls are also known to show a higher incidence of health problems, including a higher risk of obesity, type 2 diabetes and depression, independent of sleep disturbance. The full reasons for this are not understood.[168]

The influence of circadian rhythm in relation to fitness, nutrition, and sleep will be further discussed in the chapters that follow, but it is helpful to highlight a typical description of timing here. Our understanding of chronobiology and the influence of circadian rhythms is best for Larks and Third Birds; we know less about how Owls may be affected, although from a cognitive perspective it is reasonable to expect that the timings would be reversed.

## Fatigue, Ultradian Rhythms, and Scheduling Breaks to Optimise Performance

Fatigue, be it mental or physical, is experienced by us all across various settings. In the workplace it is extremely common, and its causes are multifactorial. Fatigue due to sleep deprivation is discussed in chapter 17, but fatigue is not just related to sleep deprivation. The rates at which people fatigue in specific tasks differ significantly, and this is partly related to our training and experience, our health and well-being, and our mindsets. Other factors including our chronotypes and the environment (e.g., lighting, noise, and ambient temperature) also play important roles. *All forms of fatigue start long before we realise we are losing our edge*, and hence planning ahead to prevent this is essential. This not only relates to scheduling of our activities but planning breaks from those activities too.

Whereas circadian rhythms have a twenty-four-hour cycle, there are other physiological 'mini-rhythms' that are relevant to performance. **Ultradian rhythms** are shorter, recurrent cycles across twenty-four hours. They include extra rhythms relating to mental arousal, appetite, mood, and release of some hormones (e.g., growth hormone), and their durations vary depending on the specific element involved. For example, mental arousal doesn't just follow an overall circadian rhythm, it ebbs and flows in mini (ultradian) rhythms too, which is of relevance in task performance and taking breaks. Leonardo da Vinci reportedly worked in such ultradian cycles, taking a break to sleep for twenty minutes every four hours. However, most research indicates that cycles relating to task performance are much shorter; optimal focus can be maintained for around ninety minutes. It has long been recommended that this should influence the timing of breaks, so each four-hour cycle is split into two performing blocks, each of ninety minutes duration with twenty-minute breaks on either side.[169]

In addition to pursuing a focus/rest cycle, additional micro-breaks can also be useful to some. These last just a few minutes and might involve brief social interaction (e.g., a short chat with a colleague), relaxation (e.g., stretching, looking out the window), or focusing on something else (e.g., reading the news or surfing the net). Such approaches can help

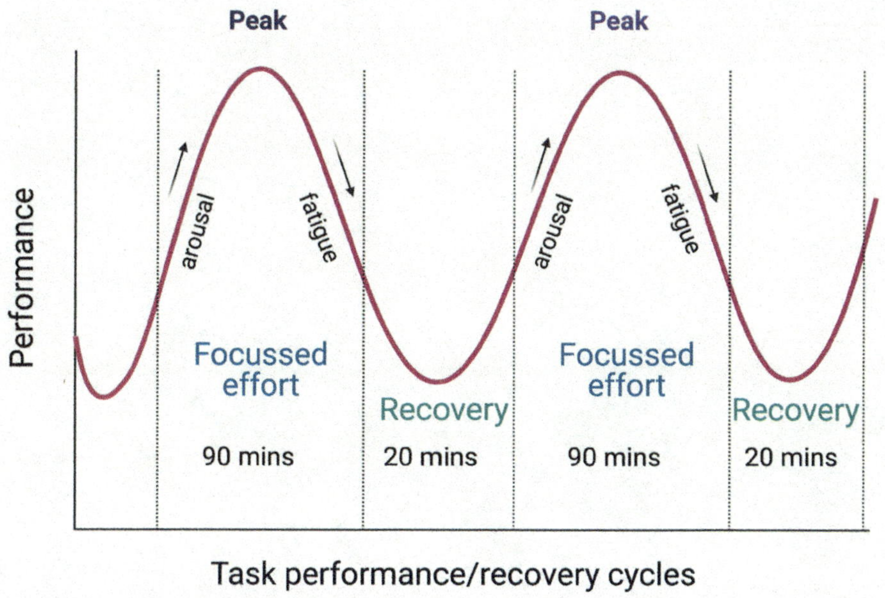


**Figure 12.3** The focus/recovery task performance cycle.

cognitive function, improve mood, and help the individual to feel more engaged with the work they are doing. Adding nutrition – e.g., snacks or caffeine – does not seem to confer added benefit. Micro-breaks seem most effective in those who start with relatively low engagement with the work they are doing and make less impact on those who are most engaged from the outset.[170]

## Key Messages:

- There are three principal chronotypes: Owls, Larks, and Third Birds.
- Establishing one's chronotype can have a major effect on performance through scheduling of activities to do the right things at the right time.
- Ultradian rhythms and the timing of breaks is also important to performance optimisation.

# 13

# Fitness

*If we could give every individual the right amount of nourishment and exercise, not too little and not too much, we would have found the safest way to health.*

**Hippocrates, 460–375 BC**

There are no surprises in saying that exercise is good for you and that it improves performance across many domains in life. There is a lot of science underpinning our understanding of exercise, the fitness it can bring, and the physiology of performing at the highest level in sport – but there are also many myths that need to be dispelled. This chapter focuses on the 'what, how, why, and when' of exercise in relation to performance: What types of exercise matter to human performance and why? How does exercise work its magic? How can we get the timing right to achieve the best effects? How do we measure and monitor fitness? These questions apply to us all. Some additional features that apply to the high performance athlete are also discussed in the next chapter, 'Fitness in the High Performance Athlete'.

## Some Basics

Regardless of what we do in life, fitness matters. But what does that really mean? ***Health-related fitness*** means protecting our bodies and minds through attaining physical, physiological, and psychological attributes that reduce the chances of diseases and death. ***Performance-related fitness*** means fine-tuning those attributes to allow us to achieve specific goals, keep stress at bay, and be able to get more out of life. It's being smart.

Physical fitness is composed of five basic elements: aerobic capacity, strength, power, balance/fine skills, and flexibility. Training can be very specific; someone can be super good in one domain and really poor in the others. If the focus is on fitness as a full package, then a programme should include all elements of fitness listed.

| |
|---|
| **Cardiorespiratory (aerobic) capacity** |
| **Muscle strength** |
| **Muscle power** |
| **Balance/neuromotor control** |
| **Flexibility** |

**Table 13.1** The five components of physical fitness. Note that many 'multimodal' forms of exercise incorporate a combination of these elements (e.g., circuits, cross-fit, and gymnastics).

### First, Move

The world has become a sedentary place, and we are suffering for it. One in four white US adults spend about 70% of their waking hours sitting, 30% in light activities, and little or no time in exercise.[171] Being sedentary is an independent risk factor for a range of diseases and premature death; those who are sedentary are twice as likely to die early. In those who sit for a total of five hours per day or more, even a burst of higher intensity activity training in the day does not mitigate the risks. Those who sit less and exercise regularly can partly mitigate the risk of their sedentary hours. For example, people who are sedentary more than four hours per day have a 40% higher risk of being obese and developing the associated diseases that result from obesity compared to those that are sedentary for less than four hours per day, but if those 'moderate sitters' exercise at least four hours per week, then those risks are significantly reduced. As a general guide, people who sit less than two hours a day are 'light sitters', people who sit two to four hours per day are 'moderate sitters', and those who sit more are 'extreme sitters'.[172]

There are various ways that sedentarism harms health, including reduced blood glucose control, leading to increased risk of diabetes, obesity, fatigue, and impaired cognition.[173] When people are sedentary, a lack of muscles activation means they waste and are replaced by fat, and the muscles that remain don't use much glucose, which is one of many contributing factors to the loss of glucose control (pre-diabetes and diabetes). Standing is a little better than sitting (especially for our spines) but really, we just have to move. Short, frequent light activity such as short walks, even if each is just five to ten minutes, spread across the day can help glucose to stay in a healthy range and to maintain insulin sensitivity. Otherwise sedentarism results in blood glucose highs and lows and the development of insulin resistance.[174]

What about the 10,000 steps mantra? Is it a myth? Sort of; it was developed as a marketing ploy by a pedometer company, but it turns out that somewhere around 7,000–9,000 steps confers major benefits to cardiovascular, mental, musculoskeletal, and metabolic health. Less can still confer significant advantages. So *don't be still: every movement counts.*

## Next, Move Quickly: Aerobic Training

What about more intensive, structured activity? That's exercise, and if it were a drug, it would be a blockbuster. There is a dose response effect, and the dose is defined by the volume we do and the intensity. We are told that to protect our health we have to do 150–300 minutes of 'moderate' or 75+ minutes of 'vigorous' physical activity a week, or a mixture of the two.[175] That's on top of keeping moving generally in the day. On a day-to-day basis we can achieve our exercise quota in ten-minute bites if we need to, though that only suits someone in an early exercise regime. It's a good place to start, but that's just for basic health.

What do *light*, *moderate*, and *vigorous* exercise intensity mean? For aerobic (cardiovascular, 'CV') work, the best definition is according to heart rate, and specifically the percentage of the heart rate capacity that the person has, called heart rate reserve (HRR). Smartwatches will calculate that. Otherwise, use Rated Perceived Exertion (RPE); a 0–10 scale is easiest.

| Exercise Intensity | HRR and RPE |
|---|---|
| **Moderate** | 40–59% HRR and RPE 5, 6 |
| **Vigorous** | 60%+ HRR and RPE 7+ |

**Table 13.2** Classification of exercise intensity based on heart rate reserve (HRR) and rated perceived exertion (RPE).[176]

| | |
|---|---|
| Take your resting heart rate (RHR) (ideally in the morning, still in bed; rest quietly for 5 minutes, count your pulse for 30 seconds, multiply by 2). Alternatively, use a smartwatch/device. | **RHR=** |
| Calculate your likely maximum heart rate (220 – age in years). | **Maximum heart rate =** |
| Subtract your resting heart rate from your maximum heart rate, which gives your heart rate reserve (HRR). | **HRR=** |
| Then decide what is a 'moderate' zone for you: (40% x HRR) + RHR. | **Moderate zone =** |
| And determine a 'vigorous' zone for you: (60% x HRR) + RHR. | **Vigorous zone =** |

**Table 13.3** How to calculate heart rates for different exercise intensities.

Above vigorous there is 'near maximal' (i.e., as close to maximum as possible). This isn't considered overall any different than 'vigorous' in terms of health benefits. 'Near maximal' intensity is a common goal in High Intensity Interval Training (HIIT), when the aim is for short bursts of exercise as high in intensity as possible, even above 89% HRR.

## Resistance training

Resistance exercise should target all major muscle groups, and can involve fixed or free weights, resistance bands, or using bodyweight. The 'dose' is described by the number of sets of repetitions. Women are significantly less likely to embrace resistance training for a range of reasons, partly because of a fear of looking too muscular. This is an unnecessary concern as, although some gains in muscle are attained, women do not naturally 'bulk up' (muscle 'hypertrophy') unless the training load is heavy. Significant gains in strength can come from changes in the ways that muscles fire.

To build muscular endurance, one or two sets of 15–25 repetitions at lower intensity (i.e., <50% of the individual's one-repetition maximum ['1RM'] effort) should be effective. For more gains in both hypertrophy and strength, two to four sets of 8–12 repetitions at 60–80% of the 1RM is recommended (i.e., moderate to hard intensity), while experienced exercisers may work at ≥80% of the 1RM (i.e., hard to very hard intensity). Rest intervals of two to three minutes between sets are most effective for achieving the desired gains.

| Benefit | CV | Resistance |
|---|---|---|
| Reduces all-cause mortality | ✔ ✔ | ✔ |
| Reduces negative cardiovascular events (e.g., heart attack, stroke) | ✔ ✔ | ✔ |
| Lowers blood pressure | ✔ ✔ | ✔ |
| Improves metabolism, increases insulin sensitivity | ✔ ✔ | ✔ ✔ |
| Improves body composition, reduces body weight/fat | ✔ ✔ | ✔ ✔ |
| Improves overall functional capacity | ✔ ✔ | ✔ ✔ |
| Protects bones | ✔ ✔ | ✔ ✔ |
| Prevents injuries | ✔ | ✔ ✔ |
| Helps balance | ✔ ✔ | ✔ ✔ |
| Reduces pain in arthritis | ✔ (avoid high impact) | ✔ |
| Improves mood | ✔ ✔ | ✔ |
| Improves energy levels | ✔ | ✔ ✔ |
| Reduces stress | ✔ ✔ | ✔ |

**Table 13.4** Evidence-based benefits of CV and resistance exercise.

**Note:** Direct comparisons have not been studied, but in general ✔ ✔ indicates greater effect than ✔. There is likely some individual variability. The point is, both modes have major benefits!

## The Principle of Training: Overload

When we exercise, we essentially 'stress' our systems, such as there is an adaptive response and, with repeated sessions over time, the body becomes better at dealing with those demands, which means it is fitter. This is true regardless of whatever element of fitness is being trained. The trick is to get the balance right, to do the right amount to progress without doing so much that the system cannot adapt, and injury, illness, or simply a lack of progress occurs. This is why planning recovery is so important – having a routine to ensure we gain from what we have done and avoid negative effects. A failure to allow recovery results in maladaptation, mental and physical fatigue, and underperformance. Individuals differ in the time they need to recover from a training session – some take hours and some need a few days, and of course that is partly influenced by the type of training session performed. Different forms of training should be spaced across the week such that all elements of necessary fitness are being addressed, but adequate recovery from each type of session is being achieved. So, if a lengthy high intensity session is performed on one day, then on the next day lower intensity work can be the focus, potentially also with a resistance training session. Table 13.5 provides an example of a weekly programme comprised of a range of different forms of training to support improvements.

| |
|---|
| Aerobic (CV) work: Higher intensity aerobic work 2–3 x week, moderate activity on 3–4 days. |
| Resistance training 2–3 x per week, on the days moderate CV is performed. |
| Warm up and cool down are both essential. |
| Add skills-specific work if appropriate. |
| One restoration day—light activity, stretching, relaxation (e.g., restorative yoga). |
| Consider incorporating more active recovery sessions where time permits. For example, on days where intensive work is done in the morning, a light intensity work, stretching, etc. might be performed later in the day. |

**Table 13.5** An example of exercise session types for a reasonably fit person across a week of fitness training.

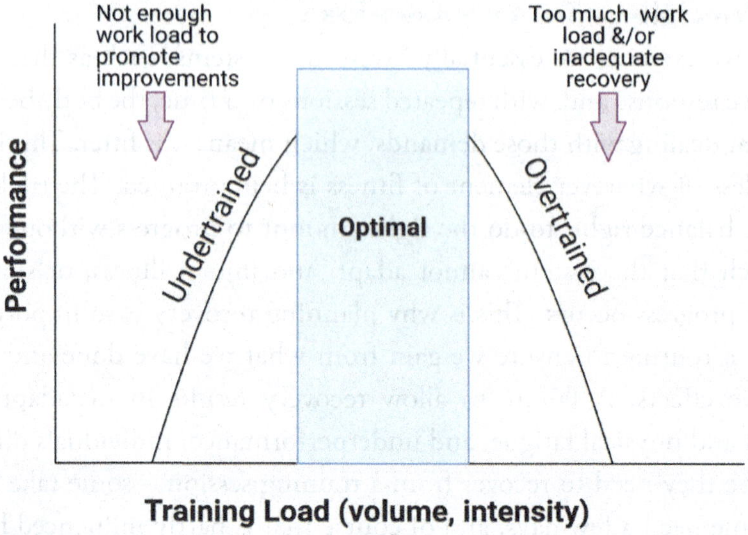


**Figure 13.1** Balancing training load to optimise gains. (Optimal load varies across individuals and changes with time and fitness.)

Getting the recipe right, ensuring effective training loads to promote fitness improvements while also ensuring adequate recovery, is an art as much as a science. The best schedules differ between individuals and may vary across time for that one individual. This is where expert support, for example from a trainer or coach, is helpful. Technologies can also help. The individual themselves will learn what they respond to and what recovery strategies apply to them, but understanding the principles is a fundamental first step.

Where training loads are excessive, or not properly interspersed with sessions that focus on other aspects of fitness and recovery, fatigue, underperformance, injuries and illness, ensue.

Fully **recovering** from an exercise session means restoring the body to a replenished state, clearing the metabolic by-products (e.g., lactate) and the inflammation resulting from the stress on the system, and allowing tissue to adapt and repair. Recovery starts *before* exercise stops, since 'cool down' (light exercise) helps to clear some of the lactate such that tissues are less stiff and sore post-exercise. Post-exercise stretching may assist with this. Hydration and 'refuelling' – ensuring suitable nutrition to rebuild energy stores – are critical and are discussed in chapter 16.

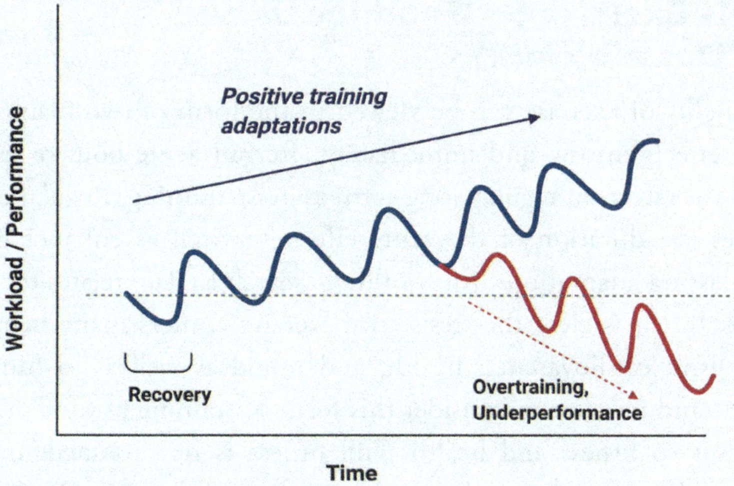


**Figure 13.2** Lack of recovery after imposed loads can result in overtraining, underperformance, illnesses, and injuries.

Other approaches are taken that aim to reduce post-exercise inflammation and muscle soreness. Popular strategies include cold water immersion (ice water baths, cryotherapy), hot water immersion, contrast (hot/cold) therapy, compression garments (e.g., socks, shorts), massage, and hyperbaric therapy. Cold water immersion soon after training may improve muscle soreness but not performance. The other measures mentioned may help some individuals feel better, but the evidence for any effectiveness otherwise is low. The use of anti-inflammatory drugs such as ibuprofen to assist with recovery is discouraged, as they are potentially harmful to health and may impair healthy tissue recovery.[177]

Warm-up at the beginning of an exercise session can also play a role in assisting recovery. Much is made about pre-training 'static' stretching, but there is little evidence that in isolation it has positive effects. However, warm-up is important. Warm-up means light exercise at progressive intensity that allows the body temperature and heart rate to gradually rise, dynamic stretching of tissues to prepare them for more loads, and shadowing and agility drills where appropriate for the sport to prepare the mind, brain, and body for the session.[178]

## Why Is Exercise So Good for Us and How Does It Work?

The benefits of exercise can be viewed in the form of two main events: (1) the effects during and immediately after an acute bout of exercise, and (2) the effects of regular, long-term exercise training. Regular exercise increases the duration of the acute effects, as well as enhancing other longer-lasting adaptations. Most of the research to date relates to aerobic exercise, but it is clear that resistance exercise confers many benefits to metabolism, cardiovascular health, and mood as well as to functional capacity, and it is fair to consider this form of training as fundamentally important to fitness and health. Full fitness is not attained unless all components of fitness are addressed, regardless of the sport involved.

A single bout of exercise reduces inflammation, and inflammation is a driver of many diseases, including cardiovascular diseases, cancer, diabetes, and dementia. Inflammation is also an important cause and effect of obesity. Exercise reduces the chances of heart attacks and strokes and protects the brain, partly through the anti-inflammatory effects, but also through a range of other mechanisms that cause the heart and arteries to adapt and work more efficiently. Light activity may help the heart, but more intensive exercise works better. As we adapt, our blood pressure and heart rates at rest and at given workloads fall, so it feels as though we are not working so hard to achieve a given workload. This is especially seen with CV training, but improvements are also seen with resistance work. Adaptations also occur across a range of organs from skeletal muscles, bones, the liver, gut, and brain, to the pancreas, where insulin is released. These changes can occur after an acute bout of exercise, but more occur with longer-term training. These adaptations are far too extensive to detail here, but some central changes that happen to the body are illustrated in figure 13.3.[179]

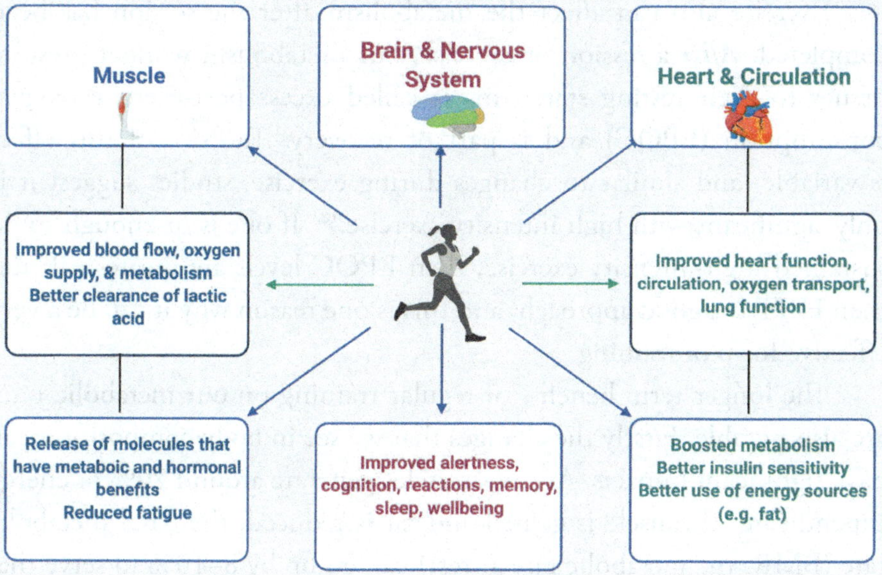


**Figure 13.3** Some of the benefits of regular aerobic exercise on the body.[180]

## Exercise, Weight, and Metabolism

There are many myths about exercise and weight loss, about the extent of calories burned and a perception that being physically active means we can eat what we want. Sadly not. Although we definitely burn more calories when active, this can easily be offset by eating a high-calorie snack. Being physically active is associated with weighing less, but it's not principally about the number of calories burned in a single session. It's more complex than that. Regular exercisers become more attuned to their bodies, make healthier lifestyle choices, have a better body composition, and tend to move a lot more in general on a daily basis. *When we feel better, we tend to live better, and we perform better.*

That is not to say that when we exercise we don't burn more calories. Of course we do, because we need more energy to do the work. If the exercise is light, then fewer calories are burned than in intense activity. Furthermore, exercise can also 'boost' metabolism. Indeed, our metabolic rates can rise ten times the resting value during sustained high intensity aerobic exercise. With lighter exercise though, these changes are unlikely.

Exercise also can affect the metabolism after the session has been completed. *After* a session of exercise, our metabolism works to restore tissues to their resting state; this is called excess post-exercise oxygen consumption (EPOC) and is part of recovery. The size of this effect is variable, and similar to changes during exercise, studies suggest it is only significant with high intensity exercise.[181] If one is fit enough to do sustained high-intensity exercise, then EPOC levels are greatest; if not, then HIIT is a good approach, and this is one reason why it can be a very effective form of training.

The longer-term benefits of regular training on our metabolic rates are also notable. Firstly the changes that we see in body composition can have significant impacts. At rest, muscles generate around 20% of energy expenditure. If muscle is gained and fat is reduced, the basal metabolic rate (BMR, the metabolic rate at rest) can go up by 8–10% to serve that extra muscle mass.[182] Increases in BMR can also be seen in those who regularly perform aerobic exercise, even without substantial changes in body composition, but again, higher intensity work is most effective in this respect.

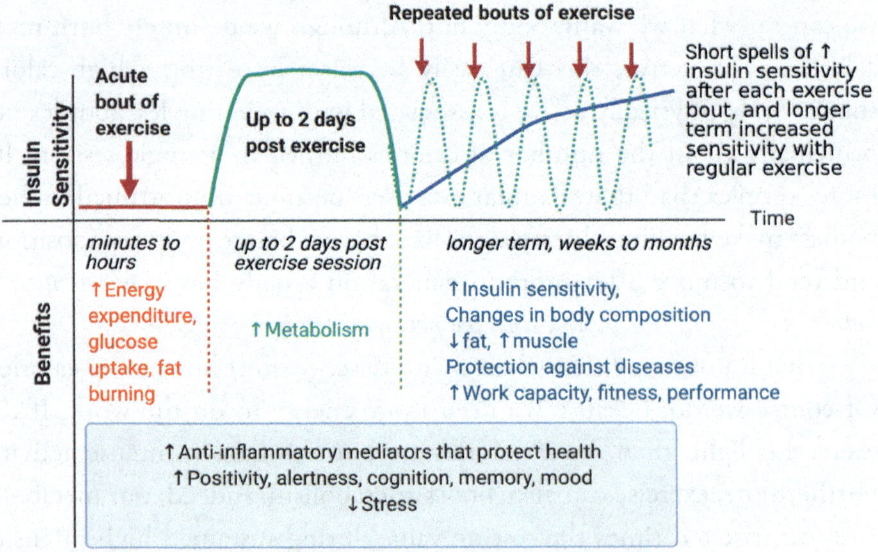


**Figure 13.4** Benefits of exercise on metabolism and performance.[183]

Exercise can change the way our bodies respond to food by improving insulin sensitivity, whereby our cells become more responsive to insulin. This reduces the likelihood of diseases including pre-diabetes and diabetes, obesity, heart disease, strokes, and dementia; and the smoother glucose control also helps to enhance energy, alertness, and cognition (see chapter 15, 'Nutrition for Us All').[184]

High intensity exercise (like HIIT, or sustained high intensity work if fit enough) and resistance training are both effective, and doing both is better. The effects on insulin sensitivity of a single exercise bout can last seventy-two hours, and regular activity leads to sustained improvement. In those who already have pre-diabetes or diabetes, lower intensities are also effective in achieving improvements in insulin sensitivity.[185]

## Back to the Brain

Physical activity has significant effects on the function and structure of the brain, and there are enormous biological and psychological benefits that are increasingly evident from scientific research. Part of the effects rely on 'neuroplasticity', which as described earlier is the brain's ability to reorganize itself by forming new nerve connections (synapses) throughout life. Neuroplasticity allows the nerve cells in the brain to compensate for injury and disease and to adjust their activities in response to new situations or to changes in their environment. Physical activity increases blood flow in the brain, and there is also a release of 'neurotrophic' (growth) factors and neurotransmitters (chemicals that relay messages) in the brain, including endorphins and serotonin, that stimulate brain function and improvements in the synapses such that the cells communicate with each other more effectively. Research has also shown that aerobic exercise can also influence 'neurogenesis', the development of new brain cells, so that there is an increase in grey matter. Remember the London taxi drivers' brains getting bigger with learning? Clearly exercise can have brain-building effects too. Cardiovascular fitness also has beneficial effects on the *function* of the brain, including enhanced cognition and executive control (adaptable thinking, planning, self-monitoring, self-control, working memory, time management, and organization).[186]

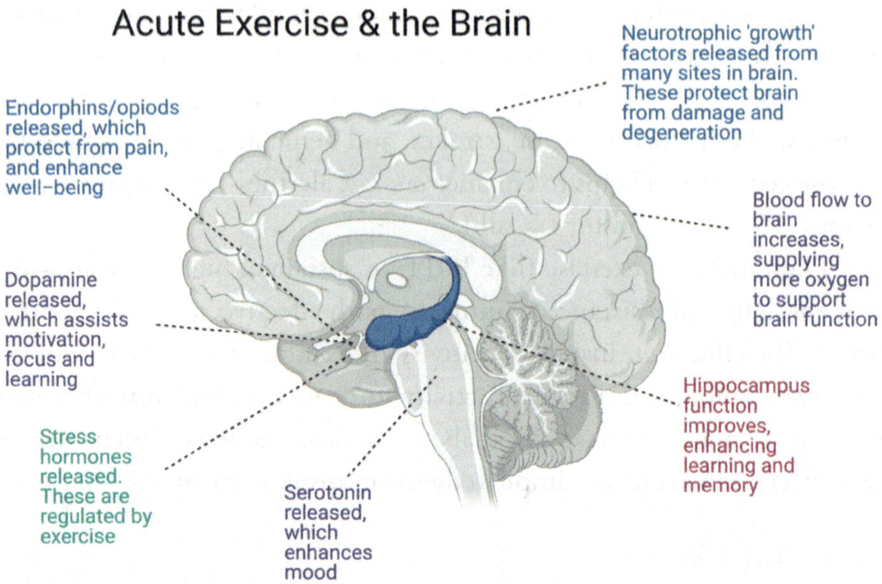


**Figure 13.5** Some of the effects of acute exercise on the brain.

Some effects of exercise on the brain are also seen in the hippocampus – a deep part of the brain that has a major role in learning and memory. There is some evidence of beneficial effects on long-term memory, learning and retention, and motor skills, partly due to effects on this area.[187]

**The mechanisms by which exercise has these effects include:**

- Increased oxygen supply through increased blood flow.
- Improvement in cardiometabolic function that improves the environment of the brain.
- Reduction in the inflammation that can cause degeneration of cells in the brain and other nerves.
- Release of chemicals such as endocannabinoids that have effects on the brain.
- Reduction in the risk of other diseases that may have direct and indirect effects on the brain.

Some of these effects arise over the course of time as fitness improves, and some occur with every acute bout of exercise, which has a positive effect on cognitive function, mood state, and stress level.

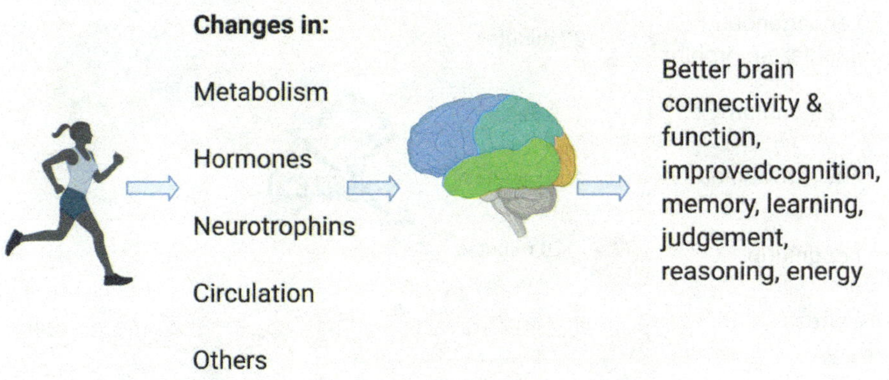


**Figure 13.6** Exercise benefits the brain through a number of mechanisms.

Although it has long been thought that moderate exercise enhances cognition but low or high intensity exercise do not, more recent research has indicated that all intensities are beneficial, but they probably vary in their effects on different areas of the brain.[188] Specifically, moderate intensity exercise may be more beneficial for executive functions whereas high intensity exercise may be more beneficial for rapid information processing.[189]

Further research has tried to address whether open-skill exercise (e.g., racket sports, hockey) differs from closed-skill exercise (e.g., running, swimming) in their effects on the brain. In one study of seventy adults in their fifties, subjects were classified according to whether they were open-skilled, closed-skilled, or irregular exercisers.[190] They then performed a working memory test while undergoing fMRI scanning. The two exercise groups, regardless of exercise modes, showed better memory scores and physical fitness performance than did the irregular exercisers. Additionally, the open-skill group exhibited greater brain activation in specific areas, including the prefrontal lobe (executive function) and hippocampus (memory, learning) than those in the closed-skill group. These findings indicate that exercise promotes cognitive health, improves working memory, and has specific positive effects on the area dedicated to executive control, and that the types of exercise may influence overall effects.

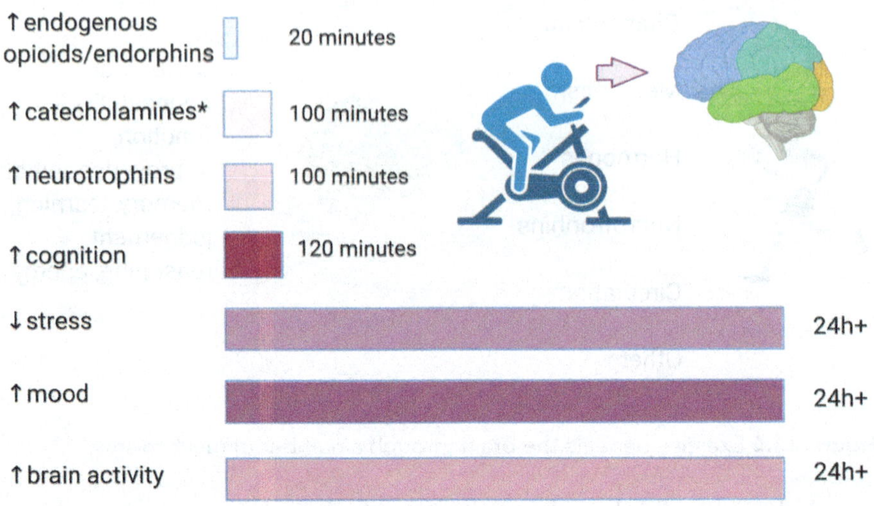


**Figure 13.7** Duration of effects after at least 30 minutes moderate to vigorous cardiovascular exercise on the brain. (More vigorous exercise seems to have greater effects.) [191]

* Catecholamines include noradrenaline and adrenaline, the acute stress chemicals, and also dopamine, the chemical messenger in the brain for pleasure, habit formation, and reward.

## What Are the Effects of Acute Exercise on Mood?

It is well established that exercise enhances well-being. It improves energy, and is associated with improved self-concept and self-esteem, self-efficacy and control, better ability to withstand stress, and positive mood. Acute exercise is one of the most effective behavioural techniques for self-regulation of mood in healthy populations, with the positive effects occurring immediately after and lasting up to one day post-exercise cessation.[192] While the 'high' that people can experience after exercise has been attributed to the release of endorphins, it is likely that other neurotransmitters like serotonin, noradrenaline, and others are also in play. Notably, endorphins release in the brain seems to occur only in high intensity exercise, but positive effects on mood can occur at lower intensities, so this confirms it isn't all about brain endorphins. In some people, high intensity may make them feel more negative, especially during higher intensity work. However, it is quite clear that most people will find exercise enhances mood, unless they are under- or over-doing it or are severely depressed.

Acute exercise not only improves mood but also reduces stress. When subjects are challenged with stressors such as complex mental arithmetic, public speaking, and other stressors after they have done a bout of acute exercise, they experience less subjective stress and reduced blood pressure during those challenges, compared to not exercising first.[193] This is a good reason for exercising prior to having to performing in a stressful situation.

Regular *inactivity* is linked to depression. Exercise is at least as effective as anti-depressants as a treatment for mild and moderate depression and can serve as an adjunct in those who do need medication.[194]

## Exercise and the Circadian Rhythm

From the chapter on chronobiology, you will know that our bodies work according to rhythms, most notably our circadian rhythm, and timing what we do and when can make a big difference to how we perform. This was also discussed more widely in chapter 8, 'Conscientiousness', but it is relevant to timing when we exercise. Our circadian rhythm not only regulates the sleep-wake cycle but also a whole range of other biological processes. It influences our metabolism, body temperature, muscle contractility, heart rate, blood pressure, and oxygen uptake into muscles, as well as various hormones including cortisol, human growth hormone, and testosterone, and (in females) oestrogen, all of which influence both our exercise performance *and* our adaptations to training. All types of exercise are affected: endurance, sprint, power, strength-related work, and flexibility.[195] These factors all play a role in influencing how we perform in exercising and the benefits we can gain. So scheduling exercise sessions to suit our circadian rhythms and the schedule of the rest of the day's activities is smart.

In general, we perform better in all forms of exercise during the second half of the day. Furthermore, because human growth hormone (HGH) is released in the late afternoon and evening and peaks overnight when we are sleeping, it is likely that our bodies will recover more effectively if we exercise in this part of the day, since HGH strongly influences tissue repair

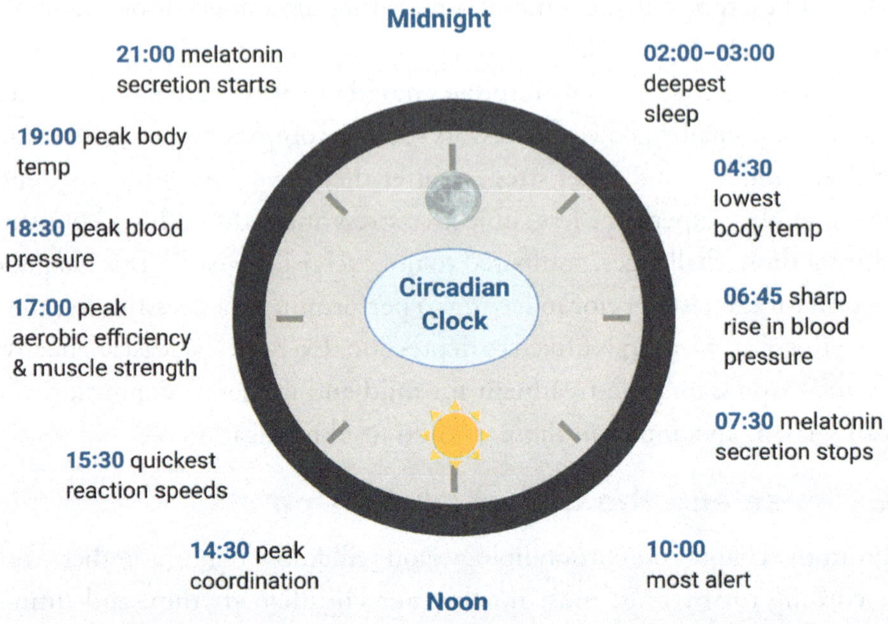


**Figure 13.8** Our circadian rhythm influences our physical performance.

and recovery. Resistance training is the form of exercise most affected by diurnal/circadian rhythms. Daytime peak muscle force is highest in the afternoon and evening (between 1600–2000) and lowest in the morning (0600–1000), with a difference between the two of up to 18% and an average difference of ~8% between performance at the different times of the day. Furthermore, we gain more strength and power if we train in the afternoon and evening.[196]

With high intensity exercise (e.g., HIIT), a similar pattern of performance and training sensitivity is seen to that of resistance exercise, peaking in the afternoon/evening and with a trough in the morning.[197]

For exercise at lower intensities (i.e., moderate intensity light exercise), the effect of the time of day on performance and response is less clear. Some studies indicate higher performance in the afternoon and evening, but the findings are not consistent.[198] This is probably because the description of moderate and endurance regimes in research studies is so wide, and it makes biological sense to expect that for most people, better performances will be in the second half of the day, so it will be the better time of day to compete, and probably to best adapt to training.

Many more world records have been set in the afternoon or evening. Even allowing for the bias of scheduling the latter stages of competition (such as semi-finals and finals) when these records are often set, performances are more likely to be better at these later times in the day.[199]

A key factor that can influence these effects in relation to circadian rhythm is our body temperature, specifically core body and muscle temperature, both of which are controlled by the brain and follow the circadian rhythm already described. These peak in the early afternoon or early evening. The effects of this temperature change in muscles include improved metabolism and contractility of the muscle, meaning it performs better during exercise. Passive warming to muscles (e.g., applying heat packs) doesn't have the same effects. Notably, oxygen uptake into muscles is better in the afternoon and evening, also contributing to enhanced performance at these times.

The influence of our circadian rhythm on sporting performance does not just relate to the physiology of our heart, metabolism, and muscles. The brain plays a big role. Our agility, motor skills, and coordination also are optimal in the later part of the day, resulting in better performance in open-skilled sports such as such as tennis and soccer.[200] It is important to bear in mind that these features of enhanced performance and better adaptations to training in the second part of the day are based on biological principles that, although applicable to us all, do not take into account our individual chronotypes. Some individuals may prefer to train and compete at times that differ from these 'optimal physiological' times. For example, Larks may simply prefer to train and compete earlier in the day.[201]

Another key consideration, of course, is the effects of exercise on sleep. Regular exercise is associated with better sleep quality through various mechanisms, including effects on body temperature, neurotransmitters, and simply making us feel more relaxed. Exercising outdoors with light exposure can also help to boost sleep. A bout of acute exercise before the late evening (i.e., before 22:00) has been shown to boost sleep quality, but exercise just before going to bed can induce a stress response that can adversely affect sleep.

Exercise can help us reset our circadian rhythm if we are sleep deprived and/or suffering jet lag, and it also can be helpful in night shift workers.[202] Up to 20% of people are engaged in night shift work. Shift workers are much more likely to develop health problems including cancer, sleep disorders, metabolic conditions (like diabetes and obesity), cardiovascular issues, and impaired mental health, largely due to the resulting dysregulation of circadian rhythm.[203]

Notably, those who travel across time zones regularly (e.g., business travellers) suffer a similar range of health issues.[204] Exercise may help to mitigate the effects by shifting the circadian rhythm and exercise during shifts (even fifteen to twenty minutes of moderate to vigorous exercise) may help to improve performance and assist in realigning sleep during the day, in addition to the typical benefits to health.[205]

Other research has shown that exercising in bright light (5,000 lux) during a break on a night shift also helps to shift the circadian rhythm.[206] Then, if there is a switch to day shifts, changing the regime accordingly may help to switch to the new demands.

## Exercise and Ageing

It is well established that regular exercise correlates with a longer life. There are many mechanisms for that, which of course relate to the reduction in risk of getting diseases, but regular activity also has an effect on our genes. There are small protein caps on our chromosomes called telomeres, and these shorten as we age. The telomeres of active people have been found to be longer, and these longer telomeres seem to account for nine years of reduced ageing of the body's cells.[207] Another example of exercise acting as a potent elixir.

## Measuring Fitness

There are measures used that are common to both health- and performance-related fitness and those that are more specific to one or the other. These are described in the tables that follow.

| Measurement | Normal/healthy | How often to measure? |
|---|---|---|
| **BMI = weight in kg/ (height in metres)$^2$** | 18.5–24.9 | BMI or weight weekly or every 2 weeks, if you are on a weight loss/gain programme |
| **Waist circumference** | <94 cm (men) and <80 cm (women) | Varies |
| **Blood pressure (BP)** | 120/80 | Every 3 months if normal; otherwise as guided by your doctor |
| **Resting heart rate** | Preferably ~ 70 but can be higher (see below) | Daily |
| **Sleep quantity** | 7–9 | Daily |
| **Sleep quality** | Score 1–10; higher is best | Daily |
| **Hydration** | Urine that is very light yellow or clear | Daily |
| **Alcohol intake** | No more than 14 units/ week | Daily |
| **Physical Activity? Amount of moderate or vigorous activity (MVPA)?** | At least 150 MVPA per week | Daily or weekly |
| **Sedentarism (time in waking hours not moving)** | As little as possible! | Daily |
| **Grip strength** | The higher the better; predictor of function and healthy ageing | Every month or so |

**Table 13.6** Basic physical health measurements that relate to both health and performance.

| | |
|---|---|
| **Full blood count** | Assess for anaemia (that can cause fatigue), ability to fight infection, others. |
| **Kidney, liver, bone profiles** | Check that organs are functioning properly |
| ***Fasting lipids** | Risk of heart and metabolic diseases, stroke |
| ***Fasting blood sugar, HbA1c** | Risk of diabetes and related conditions |
| **Iron studies** | Fatigue, energy |
| **TSH (thyroid test)** | Fatigue, energy |
| **Sex hormones** | Can decline with age and due to excessive stress or illness |
| **Vitamin D** | Muscle function, bone health, cognition, and immune status |

**Table 13.7** Basic blood tests that relate to health and performance (to be interpreted by a physician).

Note: There are other blood tests that an expert may wish to see that are specific to the situation.

| Fitness Component: Aerobic | |
|---|---|
| *Resting heart rate (beats per minute) | Low in aerobic fitness: endurance athletes can be 35 bpm. Decreases with increasing aerobic fitness. Increases suddenly in illness, under-recovery, or overtraining. |
| *Heart rate recovery | Faster recovery of heart rate after exercise indicates better aerobic fitness. |
| *Maximum oxygen uptake (VO2max) | Higher indicates more aerobically fit. Maximum test is performed in lab but estimates from wearable devices can give accurate estimates. |
| *Heart rate variability (HRV) | Greater HRV is associated with higher fitness levels. However, although many tools are available that measure this, algorithms are still not clear and the true meaning of HRV in a practical performance setting has yet to be fully established. The same issues apply to using HRV for stress and recovery. |
| Perceived exertion at a given workload | Perception of effort drops as fitness improves. Can also be used to monitor effects of resistance training. |
| Various field tests | Example: Beep test, to give estimates of VO2max |
| **Fitness Component: Strength & Others** | |
| 1 Repetition Maximum (1 RM) | The maximum weight that can be lifted once by one or more muscles (e.g., 1 RM biceps curl). |
| There are many other tests of performance-related fitness, most of which can be performed in homes or gym-based settings. These include test of balance, agility, reaction times, flexibility, etc. | |

**Table 13.8** Examples of performance-related fitness tests.

*Can be measured using wearable devices.

| Age | Poor | Fair | Average | Good | Excellent |
|---|---|---|---|---|---|
| **30s** | <39 | 39–41 | 42–48 | 49–51 | >51 |
| **40s** | <36 | 36–38 | 39–45 | 46–48 | >48 |
| **50s** | <34 | 33–39 | 37–43 | 44–46 | >46 |
| **60s** | <30 | 30–32 | 33–39 | 40–42 | >42 |
| **70s** | <28 | 28–30 | 31–37 | 38–40 | >40 |

**Table 13.9** Cardiovascular fitness: Maximum oxygen uptake (VO2max) standards in the male general population. [208]

| Age | Poor | Fair | Average | Good | Excellent |
|---|---|---|---|---|---|
| **30s** | <30 | 30–32 | 33–39 | 40–42 | >42 |
| **40s** | <28 | 28–30 | 31–36 | 37–39 | >39 |
| **50s** | <26 | 26–28 | 29–34 | 35–37 | >37 |
| **60s** | <22 | 22–24 | 25–30 | 31–33 | >33 |
| **70s** | <22 | 22–24 | 25–30 | 31–33 | >33 |

**Table 13.10** Maximum oxygen uptake (VO2max) standards in the female general population. [208]

## Measuring Recovery and Readiness

Knowing how well an individual has recovered from exercise and their 'readiness' to train and perform is a common dilemma, and a challenging area. The two are not the same: a person may be fully recovered but still not ready for an event. The tech world is full of tools with a unique selling point of dictating whether a person is fully recovered from the activities of the day before, and the products available are no doubt improving and offer significant potential, but they remain lacking in insight into the complexity of these areas. Currently there is no tool that accurately, reliably, and consistently dictates whether a person is 'recovered' nor whether they are 'ready' to take on the challenges of the day ahead. Training, nutrition, sleep, health status, mood, co-existing stresses, environments, and individuality of responses to such things means that readiness in particular is difficult to measure with a passive tool.

*Physical recovery* can be assessed through testing such as strength, power, flexibility and a lack of soreness. *Physical readiness* incorporates these elements plus a lack of injury and illness. *Physiological recovery* can be indicated by a stable resting heart rate. *Physiological readiness* is a step beyond this, and it takes into account illness, sleep, environment, stress, and mood. Psychological recovery can be assessed by simply feeling 'up for it' the next day. *Psychological readiness* means being psychologically ready for the task at hand, fully prepared to meet the challenges.

It is not too surprising then that no tool worn on a wrist, phone, or anywhere else can dictate whether the whole person is ready for a specific event. However, the individual can work through a checklist incorporating such criteria to assess their recovery and readiness status. In truth, most of the time we are not 100% ready for anything – but using the information given here will at least help to move things in the right direction.

## Conclusions

Physical activity, exercise, and fitness are all fundamental ingredients to performing in any domain in life. This is an immense topic, is critical to vitality, and deserves its prominent place in any discussion of human performance. As with all the other major elements of performance that are described in this book, the aim of this chapter has simply been to lay the foundations, the basic truths, to empower you, the reader, to explore the subject and its opportunities further.

### Key Messages:

- Regular exercise and fitness have amazing effects on our bodies and our brains and is imperative to health, well-being, cognition, and performance.
- Keep moving throughout the day.
- Aim for a minimum of 150 minutes per week of moderate to vigorous exercise.
- A good fitness programme addresses all elements of fitness: aerobic, strength/power, flexibility, balance/coordination.
- Any fitness regime should be enjoyable and fulfilling.
- Managing sleep and nutrition is important to aid recovery from any exercise session.
- Monitoring of exercise intensity and progress and recovery can be aided by using simple technology tools.

# 14

# Fitness in the High Performance Athlete

Although the principles of fitness described in the previous chapter apply to us all, there are some additional features that relate to elite athletes that give insight into the levels of fitness achieved compared to the general population, the role of physical fitness in performance at the elite level, and the balance of health versus performance-related fitness that can raise challenges.

High performance ('elite') athletes represent just a tiny fraction of one percent of the population. They are extraordinary individuals. Consider the London Marathon, which involves approximately 45,000 runners, who in themselves generally represent the fittest end of the general population. Of these, there is just a total of ~200 men and women in the two 'elite' groups. Within each of the elite groups, it is not unusual for there to be a massive 25% difference in performance times between the fastest and slowest runners in the elite pack. For example, in the 2009 London Marathon, the fastest time in the men's race was 2:05:10, the slowest time in the elite pack was 2:36:11. The average time for non-elite males to run the London Marathon is between 4:15 and 4:30.

Over the years, the nature of elite sport has been completely transformed; it is very big business, the stakes are often very high, and the pressures on the individual athlete (and their support team) are often great. The physique and the physiology of these champions have also changed. In 1950 less than 2% of NBA players were over seven feet in height. Fifty years later that figure was 12%. In the 1970s it was highly unusual for a NFL linebacker to weigh as much as 250 pounds. In 1994 weighing over 300 pounds was becoming the norm, and by 2014 many were closer to 335 pounds. In the early twentieth century, the average BMI of a sprinter was 20.5 $kg/m^2$; in the early twenty-first century it had risen to 24 $kg/m^2$. The world record for sprinting 100 metres has declined from 10.8 seconds (in 1891) to 9.58 (by Usain Bolt in 2009). In contrast, marathon runners have gotten lighter, having declined from an average BMI of 22 $kg/m^2$ to 20 $kg/m^2$ over the same time frame. While many of these changes may lead to better short-term performances in sport, the risks in some such as rugby are becoming greater due to the size and power of players involved.

## Markers of Fitness to Perform

Huge efforts are rightly made to study the physiology of champions, to ascertain what predicts their performances. There are many other examples of the physical attributes that elite athletes must attain to 'be in the game'. Elite sprinters, for example must have super-fast reaction times to the start gun to have any chance of a good performance. Reaction times of 0.166 seconds are reported in this group; consider this in the context of a blink of an eye, which takes 0.1–0.4 seconds.

Endurance (closed-skill sport) athletes are much easier to study than are those in open-skilled sports such as team ball sports or golf and tennis. The physiological factors that predict the performance of endurance athletes such as marathon runners relate to their ability to transport oxygen to their exercising muscles (VO2max), their ability to clear the by-products (e.g., lactic acid) produced in those muscles during intensive exercise (lactate threshold), and their running economy (their efficiency at using oxygen in moving at a specific speed).

The ability to reach such extreme levels of fitness (i.e., 'trainability') is partly genetically influenced, and this likely varies with the attribute in question. Much is made of the concept of trainability when the subject of 'talent identification' is discussed. Undoubtedly, genetics do play a role in how our bodies respond to intensive training and skillset acquisition, and the resilience to such heavy workloads. But while the nature versus nurture debate continues, the reality is that nurturing and supporting customised and safe training are key. Most high performance athletes have been training in their sport since early childhood and have physiologically and physically adapted to high loads of training. For example, endurance athletes undertake approximately twenty-four hours of endurance training per week for forty-five weeks of the year, for an average of fifteen years. Young 'elite' tennis players will commonly have reached their 10,000 hours of deliberate practice by the time they are fifteen or sixteen years old, and this is not unusual for an athlete in any individual or team sport.

The effects of such intensive training, particularly in those who are engaged in close-skilled sports (e.g., running, swimming, road cycling), are reflected in their markers of physical fitness. For example, elite endurance runners (male and female) typically have maximum aerobic capacities ('VO2max') of 70–85 ml/kg/min. Those in women are generally lower than men by at least 10%. Compare this to reference standards for the general populations, described in table 13.10 in the previous chapter.

Elite endurance athletes also exhibit other extreme physical and physiological features. Elite rowers, for example, may have lung capacities of nine litres, compared to around six litres in the healthy general population. The composition of muscles, the types of fibres present, is also different in elite athletes. Endurance athletes have significantly more slow-twitch endurance fibres than the general population, and power/sprint athletes have significantly more fast-twitch fibres. This is largely genetically determined, but these fibres can be significantly influenced by training.[209] Furthermore, greater abilities to tolerate difficult conditions are also seen. For example, greater abilities to tolerate hyperthermia (high body temperature) and higher levels of dehydration during an event

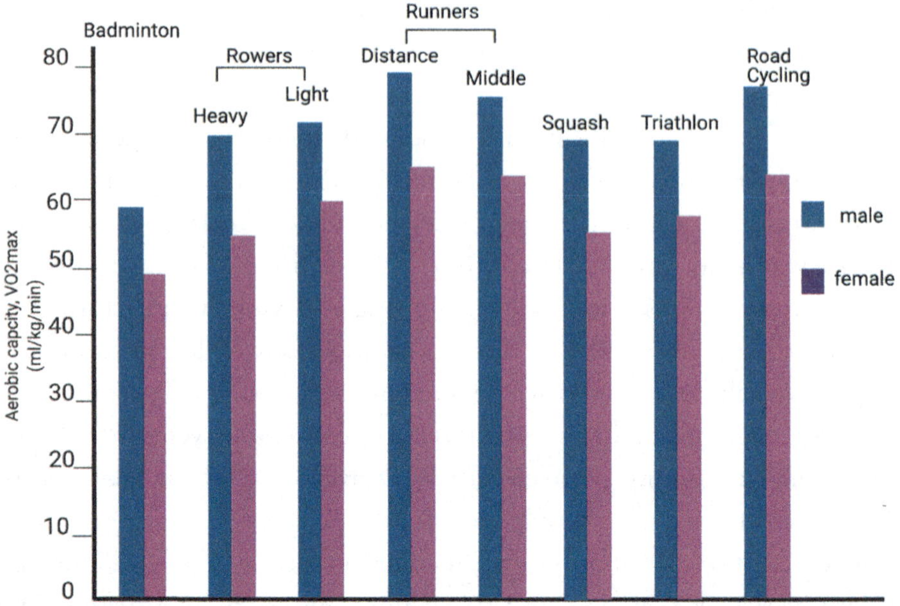


**Figure 14.1** Typical aerobic capacities (VO2max) of elite athletes in different sports.

compared to others is seen in some successful endurance runners who perform in the heat.[210]

## Multi-Skilled, Open-Skilled Sports

Moving beyond closed-skill sports, defining 'fitness' can become more challenging. Maximal power is the strongest fitness-related attribute in sports such as American football (regardless of position), rugby, and racket sports.[211] Open-skilled sports where extreme reaction speeds are especially necessary are fencing, badminton, and boxing. Badminton played at an elite level is one of the fastest sports on the planet, and the badminton shuttlecock is the fastest moving object in sport, with a world record speed of 493 km/h. Compare this to a golf ball at 339.6 km/h and tennis ball at 263.4 km/h.[212] Endurance, power, flexibility, fine motor skills, and reaction times are inherent features of performing well in badminton. Consider first the necessity for plyometric strength, to generate power to achieve high vertical jumps to smash the shuttlecock. The jump heights demonstrated by the top players, especially males, are in the highest categories (see table 14.1). Measure your own, and compare!

| Rating | Males (cm) | Males (in) | Females (cm) | Females (in) |
|---|---|---|---|---|
| Excellent | >70 | >28 | >60 | >24 |
| Very good | 61–70 | 24–28 | 51–60 | 20–24 |
| Above average | 51–60 | 20–23 | 41–50 | 16–19 |
| Average | 41–50 | 16–19 | 31–40 | 12–15 |
| Below average | 31–40 | 12–15 | 21–30 | 8–11 |
| Poor | 21–30 | 8–11 | 11–20 | 4–7 |
| Very poor | <21 | <8 | <11 | <4 |

**Table 14.1** Vertical jump height reference standards.

Beyond single 'simple' fitness markers, badminton is a good example of the complexity of other fitness prerequisites for competing at top level. It is not just simple reaction times that matter, but also choice-reaction times, where a choice needs to be made as to how to proceed – for example lunging forward to the net or pushing backwards towards the back of the court. 'Perceptual-cognitive expertise,' whereby the player knows precisely where and when to look to gather key information to anticipate what will happen, allows the player to execute the right responses in split second times and is critical to high performance.[213] Such skills are fundamental components of performance not only in badminton but also in any racket and/or ball sport. Essential as these elements of fitness are, they are difficult to measure routinely, but undoubtedly advances in performance testing technologies will assist.[214]

## Extraordinary Fitness Is Just the First Step

The chances of success in elite sport are very small. Firstly, considering talented young people, those in academy or other high performance programmes do not go on to become professional athletes. For example, only 0.5% of the 1,200 footballers in England's soccer academy system become professionals. The attrition rate across most sports is extremely high, mostly due to injury, illness, stress and negative pressures, loss of passion and motivation, inadequate support and mentorship, family circumstances, and insufficient development of skills.

Those who do 'survive' to become elite athletes as adults in any sport must possess physical characteristics, extreme physiological adaptations, and exceptional skills that are critical to performing well at the highest level. In truth though, they only get the athlete as far as having an *opportunity* to succeed; they help to get the individual over the threshold to compete at the highest level. Then it is up to other factors, the Six Keys, that determine success.

These Six Keys that determine whether the athlete achieves such extreme physical and physiological attributes, but also how they then execute the performance on a given day. The journey to any event is demanding and full of challenges that will defeat many. There are many factors that determine who will be a champion: passion for the goals, perseverance with training (often with setbacks along the way), intrinsic motivation, self-awareness when preparing and managing challenges, conscientious planning of training, gaining knowledge, focusing on deliberate practice, careful self-management, self-efficacy in ensuring the right support is there, and executing the right behaviours relating to vitality – sleep, nutrition, training, recovery, staying in a positive mindset, and avoidance of energy-sapping distractions.

*Being your best is not so much about overcoming the barriers other people place in front of you as it is about overcoming the barriers we place in front of ourselves. It has nothing to do with how many times you win or lose. It has no relation to where you finish in a race or whether you break world records. But it does have everything to do with having the vision to dream, the courage to recover from adversity and the determination never to be shifted from your goals.*

**Kieren Perkins, Olympic Gold Medalist, swimming**

# 15

# Nutrition for Us All

Nutrition is central to health, well-being, and performance, affecting every component of these domains. 'Nutrition' applies not just to our energy supply but to the supply of a range of nutrients that can have a range of beneficial effects. 'Good nutrition', 'healthy foods', 'sensible eating' are all terms that are considered by many in a negative context, as too much like hard work, not enjoyable in a busy world with constant access to addictive 'hyperpalatable' (high sugar and fat) foods that are often eaten on the move as snacks, with little focus on structured eating times. Unfortunately, information about nutrition is often confusing. In a poll of over 1,000 Americans asked, 'Which is harder: figuring out what you should and shouldn't eat, or figuring out how to do your own taxes?' 52% said knowing what to eat was more challenging.[215]

Good nutrition is a lot more satisfying than bad nutrition, and since it is so critical to performing well, time is well spent in gaining an understanding of what we should eat, how much, when, and why. It is a topic with such a wide scope that only a succinct overview that relates to performance can be provided here. The focus is on essential body composition, energy balance, metabolism, the true dangers of sugars, and

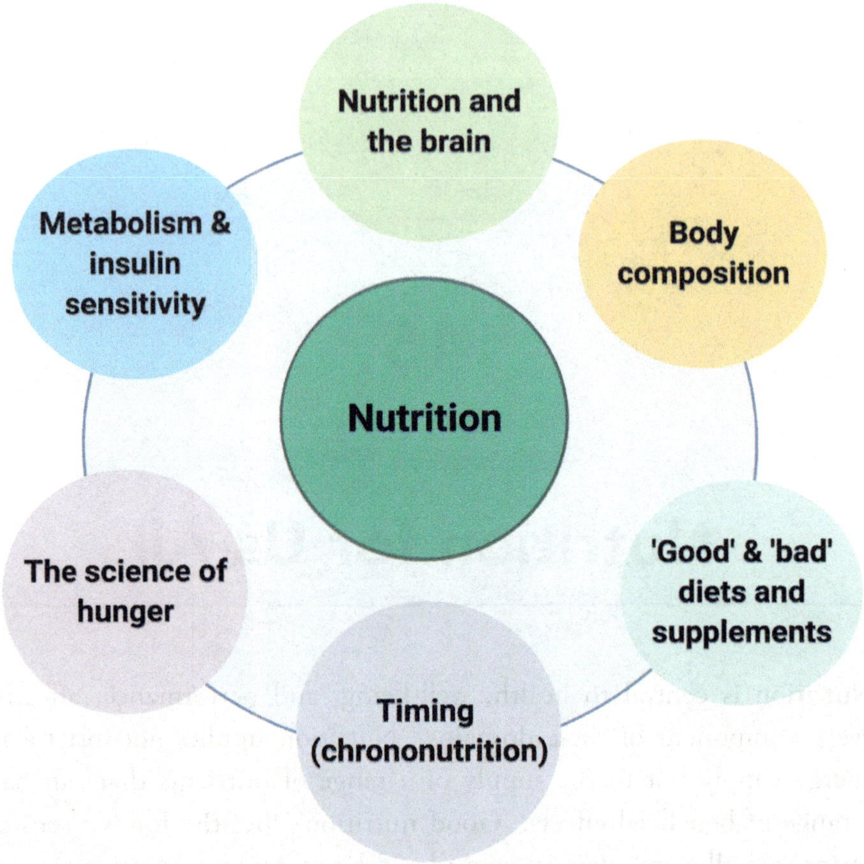


**Figure 15.1** Important considerations relating to nutrition for performance.

the need for balanced healthy nutrition for vitality. Nutrition for more serious athletes is also discussed in the next chapter.

## The Why and How of Nutrition: Energy Balance, Hunger, and Metabolism

Any sensible introduction to nutrition for vitality and performance should start with a review of body composition and energy needs.

### Body Composition

Body composition is an index of physical fitness, and it expresses the amount of muscle, fat, bone, and water that forms the body's habitat. Two bodies that weigh the same can look completely different depending on the lean (non-fat) tissue they have. There are different ways of measuring body composition, including skin folds measurement by a trained individual (to measure body fat) and DEXA (dual energy absorptiometry) scanning (which measures total body composition), both of which can give accurate results. Other approaches (e.g., bod pods) are less reliable. At home, bioelectric impedance analysis on 'smart scales' is also widely available, and although less accurate than expensive tools like DEXA, this can be helpful to chart progress regularly, providing that high quality smart scales are used and measurements are always taken under the same conditions (undressed, same time of day, hydrated, before/after food). However as with all tech products, be selective and be wary of duds.

Body mass index (BMI; weight [kg]/height [in metres]$^2$) gets a lot of bad press in terms of its usefulness in some people, because athletes with a lot of lean muscle have high BMIs. However, it is still useful for many, and in combination with other measures like waist circumference, it's a good start. BMI and waist circumference tools are given in the appendix at the end of the book.

| Category | BMI |
|---|---|
| Underweight | <18.5 |
| Normal | 18.5–24.9 |
| Overweight | 25–29.9 |
| Obese | 30 and above |

**Table 15.1** Body Mass Index (BMI) categories.[216]

Our body fat includes essential body fat to maintain life and healthy functions as well as storage fat, which is the type that many people have in excess. It is possible to have too little body fat, and this can threaten a person's health. But more commonly, people have too much fat, and this has different consequences on health depending on where it is stored.

Essential fat is located in our bone marrow and also in necessary amounts to protect our brain, nerves, and organs. The types we have too much of is storage fat – both fat under the skin and visceral fat (around organs). Although both types of storage fat in excess are dangerous to our health, the visceral fat is more of a threat and is strongly linked to heart disease, diabetes, and dementia.

| Body fat | Male | Female |
|---|---|---|
| **Essential fat** | 3–5% | 10–14% |
| **Total fat in athletes** | 6–14% | 14–21% |
| **Total fat in fit people** | 14–18% | 21–25% |
| **Total fat in the average western population** | 18–25% | 25–32% |
| **Total fat in obese people** | >25% | >32% |

**Table 15.2** Percentage body fat in different groups.

## Energy Balance and Calories

Energy balance (i.e., energy intake versus expenditure) is of course a central part of overall energy management. When it comes to calories, everyone fusses about them, and some obsess about them. They are part of energy balance of course, but the topic of calories is just one aspect of how to eat intelligently and enjoyably. It may be true that 'a calorie is a calorie', but some calories are better than others and indeed are metabolised differently depending on when they are ingested. Our metabolism and storage of fuels is largely influenced not only by energy-in versus energy-out, but also by the *timing* of energy intake and *type* of foods we eat. The energy produced from foods depends on how we eat it, what we eat with it, and how we digest it.

## Calculating Calorie Needs

Calculating calorie needs on the basis of our energy expenditure can be difficult. Wearable devices like bands and watches may give us a calorie consumption record, but as yet none of these are accurate – they at best give you ballpark figures. There are algorithms to make this calculation ourselves, but they are based on estimates depending on activity category rather than the exact amount of activity that day, personalised to that individual. Still, they are quite useful if one has a fairly consistent schedule.

## Understanding Our Metabolism

There are three main elements to the energy our body burns each day: (1) the energy we burn just to stay alive and function at rest (basal metabolic rate, BMR); (2) the energy we use in being active (exercise thermogenesis); and (3) the energy we use to digest food (dietary thermogenesis, around 10% of total). BMR can be calculated using various equations; the Henry Equation is frequently used, although there are others.[217]

Total calorie needs to maintain weight can be calculated by multiplying BMR by the appropriate activity factor, as shown in table 15.4.

| Age | Male | Female |
|---|---|---|
| 18–30 | 16 x weight (kg) + 545 | 13.1 x weight (kg) + 558 |
| 30–60 | 14.2 x weight (kg) + 593 | 9.74 x weight (kg) + 694 |
| 60+ | 13.5 x weight (kg) + 514 | 10.1 x weight (kg) + 569 |

**Table 15.3** Calculation of BMR using the Henry Equation.

| Activity Level | Calories |
|---|---|
| Sedentary (little or no exercise) | BMR x 1.2 |
| Lightly active (light exercise 1–3 days per week) | BMR x 1.375 |
| Moderately active (moderate exercise 3–5 days per week) | BMR x 1.55 |
| Very active (vigorous exercise 6–7 days per week) | BMR x 1.725 |
| Extra active (very strenuous exercise 6–7 days per week or physical job or twice daily training) | BMR x 1.9 |

**Table 15.4** How to calculate total daily calorie needs.[218]

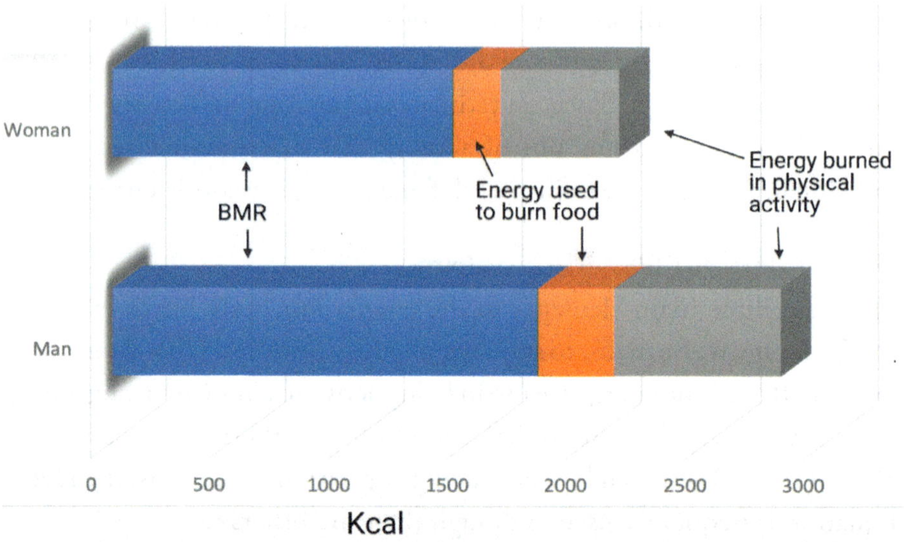


**Figure 15.2** An example of the way individuals burn energy through their BMR, dietary thermogenesis, and physical activity.[219]

Apart from serious endurance athletes or those with a heavy manual job, our BMR accounts for most of the energy we burn. It is therefore not surprising that exercise, while linked to body composition and some weight loss, does not directly burn so many calories that we can eat whatever we want. However indirect effects on energy balance can be significant, for example, through effects of activity on our insulin sensitivity. Furthermore, when we exercise, we feel better, we sleep better, etc. Success breeds success.

Our BMR depends on a few things. It is partly genetically programmed, and we are all programmed differently, so there is no point in planning our intake according to what works for someone else. BMR is faster when the body composition is one with more lean tissue (muscle) and less fat. It slows by about 2–3% per decade from our twenties; that's partly because we often gain fat, which is linked to a slower BMR. Women burn less calories than men, and their BMR can speed up by as much as 10% in the first phase of their menstrual cycles.

How does diet affect our BMR? Very low calorie diets can result in the BMR slowing by as much as 20% because the body goes into 'survival in starvation' mode. What about foods that are said to 'speed up your metabolism', like chillies, caffeine, and other spices? If they do, the effect is so small and transient it is not worth bothering with.

As indicated, there are other ways of increasing our metabolic rates. Gaining muscle is effective. The estimated metabolic rate of muscle is 10–15 kcal/kg/day, and the metabolic rate of fat is in the region of 4.5 kcal/kg/day. Note, though, that the combined energy expenditure of your brain, liver, kidneys, and heart makes up about 80% of your total BMR. These organs have a metabolic rate that is 15–40 times greater than their equivalent weight of muscle and 50–100 times greater than fat tissue![220]

What about the effects of exercise on our resting metabolism? During and immediately after exercise (particularly high intensity exercise), our metabolism is accelerated; that's 'exercise thermogenesis', and it is related to post-exercise oxygen consumption, as discussed in the previous chapter. Exercise also positively influences insulin sensitivity, which adds to the effects on our body composition, which is also aided by regular resistance training.

## Insulin Sensitivity

Insulin sensitivity has been mentioned several times in this book, illustrating its importance to our metabolism and performance, because it massively influences how our bodies manage and store our friend and foe, glucose. Insulin is released by the pancreas and triggers receptors in cells in all tissues (e.g., muscle, brain), making them take up glucose when supplied to them. The receptors become less sensitive if there is glucose around a lot of the time, such as with regular snacking, high simple carbohydrate diets, or overeating in general. Then the glucose doesn't get taken up by the cells as it should be and instead goes somewhere else for storage – and that's fat cells, anywhere around the body including around body organs (visceral fat). More glucose means more insulin, and that triggers hunger and fatigue, poor performance, more fat, and ultimately obesity, diabetes, and cognitive decline.

Most modern diets are carb overloaded, and in particular with high glycaemic index carbs, which are the worst for insulin spiking. **Glycaemic Index (GI)** is an indicator of how quickly an insulin spike will occur after ingestion, and how much of a sugar 'high' and 'low' follows. It is a useful tool in making food choices. **Glycaemic *Load*** (GL) uses the index to calculate how much a portion of a food will raise blood glucose.

**GL = (GI x available grams of carbohydrate in the portion) /100**

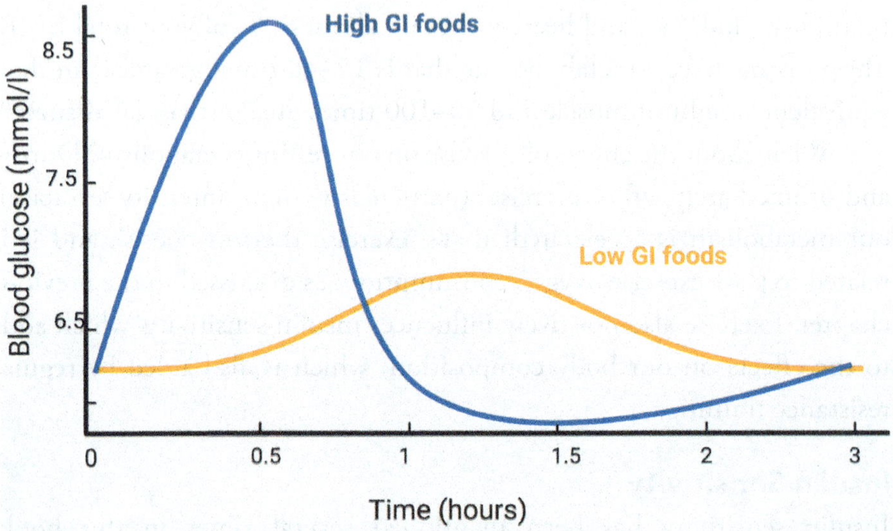


**Figure 15.3** How blood glucose spikes and falls with food of low and high GI values.

| Level | Glycaemic Index | Glycaemic Load |
|---|---|---|
| **Low** | <55 | <10 |
| **Medium** | 58–69 | 11–19 |
| **High** | >70 | >20 |

**Table 15.5** Glycaemic index and load ranges.

## Nutrition and the Brain

For our brain to function well, it constantly needs energy. The BMR of the brain is a phenomenal 240 kcal/kg/day, the highest of any organ, and receiving an optimal energy supply is top priority over other organs such as skeletal muscle.

The body's environment has a significant impact on the brain. Bad diets are pro-inflammatory, and so is carrying extra body fat. This inflammation causes widespread tissue damage, including to the brain, with the potential for causing damage to brain cells, harm to its wiring system, and impairment of a number of functions, including cognition, memory, learning capacity, emotions, and motor function. Like other tissues, the brain is also an insulin sensitive organ, and insulin affects important brain mechanisms that underlie eating behaviours, food intake, and the body's whole metabolism. People who develop insulin resistance in the brain (for the same reasons that they develop it elsewhere) are less successful in losing weight in a lifestyle intervention programme and are more likely to store visceral fat.

Our brain is not only influenced by the environment of the body in general, but it is also specifically closely linked to the gut, through what is described as the ***brain-gut axis***. Within our guts there is the **microbiome**, consisting of bacteria, fungi, and viruses. There are 100,000 times the number of microbes in a single person's gut as there are people on earth! Such microbes have profound effects on our health, assisting with digestion, metabolism, weight control, detoxifying some of what we eat, regulating the immune system, and protecting us from harmful agents. On the other hand, if there is a disturbance in the microbiome, negative consequences on health from gut diseases, immune dysfunction, and brain and nerve disorders can occur. Additionally, the commonly suffered 'irritable bowel syndrome' (IBS) is likely to reflect dysfunction of the brain-gut axis.

The brain-gut axis means that the two are connected, for example through nerves and hormones (including insulin and an appetite hormone, ghrelin) that allow two-way communication. There are some obvious examples, such as when we experience emotions the brain sends

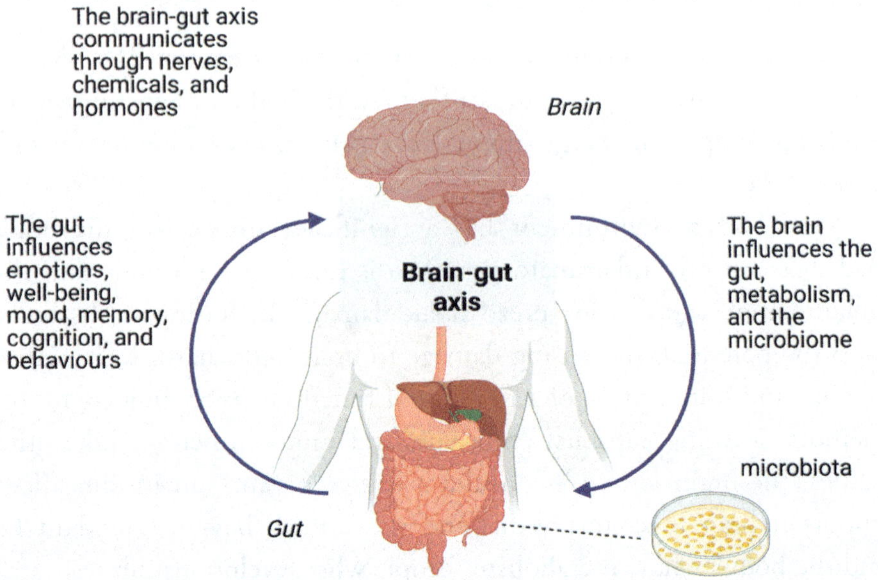


**Figure 15.4** The brain-gut axis has a major influence on how we perform.

out signals to the gut and you may experience a response – e.g., abdominal cramps when stressed; or when we see our favourite foods our tastebuds are stirred, the saliva flows, and our stomachs may grumble.

Signalling also occurs in the opposite direction. What happens in the gut is relayed to the brain. The state of our microbiome is communicated to the brain and affects our cognition, memory, emotions, learning, and other behaviours. It brings new meaning to the phrase 'go with your gut feeling'! *Anything that adversely affects the microbiome therefore affects our vitality and performance.* Those threats come from poor diets and other sources such as the use of antibiotics. People who have 'bad' microbiomes have fewer microbes and there is less diversity. This 'dysbiosis' is seen commonly in obesity.

When it comes to making food choices, nutrition plans that are good for the microbiome are those that are plant based. Probiotics are also potentially useful and are discussed further in the section on supplements later in this chapter. Approaches that are bad for the microbiome are high protein diets, fructose, saturated fats, and drugs such as antacids and antibiotics.

| Vitality component | Healthy microbiome | Unhealthy microbiome |
|---|---|---|
| Cognition | ↑ | ↓ |
| Mood | ↑ | ↓ |
| Memory | ↑ | ↓ |
| Behaviours | ✓ | ✗ |
| Inflammation | ↓ | ↑ |
| Insulin sensitivity | ↑ | ↓ |
| Metabolism | ↑ | ↓ |
| Weight control | ↑ | ↓ |
| Energy | ↑ | ↓ |
| Risk of disease | ↓ | ↑ |

**Table 15.6** Associations between components of vitality and the gut microbiome.

Carbohydrates are still important to performance, but as will be discussed further, choose carefully.

## The True Danger of Sugars and the Science of Hunger

When it comes to our health and performance, diets high in sugars are not so 'sweet' in their effects on us. Global obesity has tripled since 1975 due to excessive sugar intake and inactivity. High sugar intakes are linked to cognitive impairments, slowing of the ability of the brain to adapt and repair, memory dysfunction, lack of focus, reduced well-being, and emotional disorders such as anxiety and depression, in addition to the pro-inflammatory effects of obesity on all of the body's systems. It's no secret; sugar intake is a dangerous addiction.

**Hunger** is a complex phenomenon driven by a number of signals throughout the body and brain that tells us we *want* or we *need* to eat. The difference between 'wanting' and 'needing' means there are two types of hunger. One, '*homeostatic hunger*', is the type that is part of our survival

| | |
|---|---|
| **Biochemical effects** | • Increased inflammatory mediators that damage brain tissue<br>• Changes in dopamine and serotonin levels, which influence mood and mental health<br>• Insulin resistance in the brain, damaging to tissue and limiting effectiveness of energy supply<br>• Altered local immune function |
| **Effects on health and performance** | • Loss of control of eating behaviours and cravings<br>• Anxiety<br>• Depression<br>↓ Cognition<br>↓ Memory<br>↓ Learning<br>↓ Alertness |

**Table 15.7** Examples of the effects of high sugar intake.

mechanism. It signals that we need food for fuel. The second type of hunger is the 'I want' hunger, also called '*hedonic hunger*'. It is driven by a desire to seek pleasure from highly palatable foods. The more we eat of certain foods, the more our brain expects – craves – them. That doesn't mean pleasure isn't associated with satisfying homeostatic hunger, but it's just not the principal trigger.

At this point it is helpful to describe the two principal hormones that are particularly important to regulating our eating behaviours. The first is called **leptin** (Greek, *leptos*, meaning 'thin'). Leptin is predominantly made by fat cells and cells in the intestine. Leptin helps to controls hunger by acting on various parts of the brain, especially the hypothalamus. Here it triggers receptors in one area that inhibits hunger, and it also triggers receptors in a second area that tell us we are satisfied after eating (satiety). Since leptin is released by fat cells, higher levels are seen in obesity, but these people develop a resistance to leptin (a bit like they develop resistance to insulin too), and so the leptin stops controlling hunger.[221] Furthermore, because the brain becomes more resistant to leptin, reducing calorie intake may become ineffective in changing hunger control. Leptin has other effects on the body including acting in the hippocampus in the brain, which, you may recall, is a centre for learning and memory.[222] Leptin has positive effects on the immune system, bone health, and our hormones, and it benefits our circulation, helping to protect against atherosclerosis. Hence the impact of developing leptin resistance is very significant.[223]

The second hormone to highlight is **ghrelin**. Often called the '*hunger hormone*', it is produced by cells mostly located in the stomach. As our energy supplies run low, ghrelin is released, which acts on the pituitary gland and hypothalamus and induces appetite. Its levels are then suppressed when we eat.

In homeostatic hunger, leptin and ghrelin and other hormones in the brain play roles in balancing out hunger versus satiety. Eating nutritious foods that are high in protein, low-GI high-fibre carbohydrates, and appropriate amounts of natural fats (e.g., in olive oil, salmon, some dairy, nuts, seeds, and avocados) results in earlier satiety than foods that are high GI or highly processed.[224]

It's that simple – or it should be. But of course it isn't, because the second type of hunger, hedonic hunger, is often what governs people's eating habits. The science behind hedonic hunger, why we eat more than we need, is complex, but partly due to the brain getting very confused about what the body needs, and what will satisfy it. Following a diet with high sugar content increases cravings and reduces impulse control, lowering the ability to resist high fat/high sugar foods that perpetuate the problem. Sugar is found everywhere in the Western diet – not just in the obvious sweet foods, but also in many processed foods, bread, drinks, and sauces. Taste buds are trained to expect sweet things and are unhappy when not satisfied. The addition of sweeteners has magnified this. Hedonic hunger is often triggered by our emotions, habits, and environmental state, and it is often linked to cravings triggered by cues that may be situational, emotional, or stress related. So we are back to the challenge of habits, cues, cravings and rewards, as described in chapter 8. Only intentional habit change will address the issue in that circumstance, and this can be very challenging, because in essence sugar is an *addiction*, and addictions are very difficult to control, even in the face of negative consequences. Habit changes can only be made through planning, conscientiousness, and utilising self-effectiveness. Part of this involves retraining our tastebuds and brains to savour the true flavours of natural, healthy foods and drinks, and to derive pleasure from eating them.

Cravings can also be driven by dehydration, poor sleep, jet lag, lack of exercise, and stress. Limited sleep increases ghrelin and decreases leptin, and hunger is increased. Cravings increase too, and food choices become less healthy. Addressing sleep debt helps restore balance.

In hedonic hunger, when a craving is experienced, exercise can help, both as a form of distraction and to reduce appetite. A short intense workout is best, as this influences hormones that reduce appetite, and these hormones are related to restoring metabolic balance as a priority over replenishing energy. The same is not true for other types of workouts: low or moderate intensity activity may make us more hungry; that may be because the appetite-suppressing hormones are not released to the same extent. So it may be best to schedule these types of workouts for when we are due for a main meal afterwards anyway.

## Stress and Eating

Stress affects appetite and eating behaviours in most people. Only around 20% are unaffected. In response to stress, about 40% don't want to eat, and 40% develop hedonic hunger, 'comfort eating', seeking high fat, high sugar foods. In these people, stress encourages irregular eating patterns and hedonic overeating. This partly depends on the nature and timing of the stress. Why this happens is not clear, but it is likely to be related to effects on hormones and neurotransmitters, the brain chemicals that influence brain function. One neurotransmitter is dopamine; it is released when cortisol levels are high, and also with certain food cues, and can be linked to a triggering of compulsive behaviours.

## The 'What' of Nutrition

A protein-rich or a balanced meal results in better cognitive performance than a carbohydrate-rich meal. There are probably several mechanisms for this, but one is that carbohydrate-rich food increases brain tryptophan, which results in synthesis of serotonin in the brain and increased drowsiness.[225] Higher-carbohydrate meals also are associated with slower reaction times. Research has shown that those given a tryptophan pill felt less alert, had less vigour, and felt more fatigued. Conversely, a protein-rich meal resulted in increased levels of tyrosine, which led to increased neurotransmitter synthesis, including dopamine and noradrenaline.[226] Dopamine enhances focus, attention, and mood.

There are some basic principles that guide the content of a good nutrition plan:

- Follow the Mediterranean diet as a template.
- Avoid processed foods.
- Focus on steps towards enhancing insulin sensitivity, including reducing carbohydrates, avoiding refined sugars; instead aiming for complex carbs and low glycaemic load foods, having regular meals, and avoiding frequent snacking.

## The Mediterranean Diet

Much is made of the traditional Mediterranean diet for health, and with good reason. It is low in sugars and starch, has wholegrains, pulses, and more complex carbohydrates in the form of vegetables (green and leafy vegetables are best). The Mediterranean diet is also high in protein, and contains healthy fats. Healthy fats are those that are mono- or poly-unsaturated. Monounsaturated fats promote 'good' cholesterol (HDL) and reduce 'bad cholesterol (LDL), and can be found in some nuts (almonds, Brazil nuts, peanuts), avocado, and olive and rapeseed oils. Polyunsaturated fats such as omega-3 and omega-6 reduce the 'bad' LDL. The best source of omega-3 is oily fish (e.g., salmon, sardines, and others including cod). Omega-6 is found in rapeseed, corn, and sunflower vegetable oils, and some nuts (e.g., sunflower, walnuts, sesame seeds).

Saturated fats are the 'bad' ones and are found in fatty meat, meat products, confectionary, butter, lard, cream, ice cream, cakes, biscuits, some savoury snacks, coconut and palm oil, and cheese. This is not to say that they must be banned, but they should be kept to a minimum and certainly <20 g per day for females and <30 g per day for males.

The Mediterranean diet is associated with a reduced risk of diseases including mental health complaints, cancers, cardiovascular diseases,

<table>
<tr><th>Healthy Fats<br>(small amounts daily)</th><th>Protein</th><th>Unrefined carbs</th><th>Unlimited non-starchy vegetables</th></tr>
<tr><td>Avocado</td><td>(Meat only sparingly, once weekly at most)</td><td>Fruits (5-a day servings of fruit/ veg)</td><td rowspan="4">Lettuce, broccoli, tomatoes, peppers, onions, courgettes, peas, etc.</td></tr>
<tr><td>Unsaturated fats, oils e.g olive oil</td><td></td><td>Pasta</td></tr>
<tr><td colspan="2">Fish – twice weekly, including oily fish at least once weekly<br>Eggs<br>Some dairy/dairy alternatives e.g Soya<br>Nuts, beans, pulses</td><td></td></tr>
<tr><td></td><td colspan="2">Grains<br>Wholegrain bread</td></tr>
</table>

**Table 15.8** The Mediterranean diet.

metabolic problems such as high cholesterol and diabetes, dementia, and arthritis.[227] It is a very good example of an ***anti-inflammatory diet***. As has been discussed elsewhere in this book, avoiding things that are pro-inflammatory is key to health and performance. The Mediterranean diet is also full of **antioxidants**, which mop up damaged cells and harmful molecules in the body. There are other anti-inflammatory diets, such as the DASH diet, which is designed for those with high blood pressure.[228] The range of anti-inflammatory diets that are proposed are not far from the Mediterranean template, and the recommendation is that even if tweaked, it is the best place to start.

## Balancing Protein, Carbohydrates, and Fats

There is a lot of debate about how our diet should be structured, i.e., how much of our calories should be obtained from protein, fat, and carbs respectively.

**Protein**: Protein intake can vary from 15 to 35% of total energy intake, with higher levels being more suitable for those who are very active, training very intensively, or are in endurance or power-based sports. For those who are regularly active (around one hour per day of moderate to vigorous exercise), then mid-range is suitable. If the aim is to build muscle, it doesn't necessarily mean that very high protein intake is necessary; physical training helps the body to utilise whatever fuel it has to promote muscle growth. However, taking in protein helps the muscle to adapt and repair after training, regardless of the training type. (This is further discussed in the next chapter).

If the aim is to lose weight, many find that increasing protein helps, partly because it helps them to reduce hunger, thereby reducing the desire to reach for sugars, and it is helpful for muscle recovery after exercise. In fact, for those who need to lose weight who are also doing heavy resistance exercise, a high-protein diet while maintaining on lower calories is often recommended.

Protein is made of building blocks called 'amino acids'. We need about twenty different amino acids for health. Some foods have all of these amino acids; these are called complete protein foods. Incomplete protein foods are those that have some but not all of the amino acids we need. Leucine is a key amino acid for building muscle, and so if resistance training and muscle development are a goal, then knowing the foods high in leucine is important. High leucine foods include: chicken, fish (tuna), tofu, canned beans, milk, cheese, squash seeds, and eggs. Beef and pork are also high in leucine, but in the case of beef, red meat too often is discouraged as excessive intakes are linked to bowel cancer, heart disease, and diabetes.

Whole food sources of protein are preferred, and this can be drawn variably from the items in the Mediterranean diet. Healthy sources include: chicken, turkey, fish, cottage cheese, nuts, and eggs.

**Fats**: Around 25–35% of calories should come from healthy unsaturated fats, limiting saturated fat intake to <7% of total calories. Avoid trans fats, which are artificially created fats used to flavour foods. High fat diets do not enhance exercise performance.

**Carbohydrates**: The remainder of our diet is made up of carbohydrates. Carbohydrates are a much-needed source of energy, and many who are active will struggle on diets that are too low in carb content. Of course this depends on the activity level, exercise type, intensity, and goals. For those who exercise regularly, carefully timed carbohydrate intake helps recovery, protects our immune system, aids hormonal balance, and prevents fatigue. The point is that the carbs we eat should be predominantly low glycaemic index, high fibre carbs – not fast sugars – and timed to get the most benefit from them. (This will be discussed further in the next chapter.)

## High Protein, Low Carbohydrate Diets

It is quite clear that the foundation for eating for health and performance is ensuring healthy fats are taken in small quantities, protein intake is optimised, and care is taken about the amount and type of carbohydrates eaten.

Low carbohydrate diets, meaning those that derive <30% calories from carbs, are popular in weight loss programmes. Ketogenic diets are extremely low in carbs, typically 30–50 g/day, with a high fat intake. This induces 'ketosis', where ketones from fat become the main energy for the body and brain, instead of glucose. These diets are proposed to be beneficial in some situations including managing overweight individuals with cardiometabolic and other conditions, but there are many who do not find them suitable, and they are often not sustainable in very active individuals. There is also the risk of micronutrient deficiencies.

For those who exercise regularly, low carb diets can create challenges. It depends on the exercise, its intensity and duration, and the individual. We particularly use fat in low intensity endurance exercise, and more carbs at higher endurance exercise intensities. If we are adequately refuelled, there is about two hours of glycogen (carbs) supply in our muscles, and this is used preferentially in exercise. Ketogenic athletes burn more fat

| Type of diet | Carbohydrate | Fat | Protein |
|---|---|---|---|
| Typical Western diet | 60% | 15% | 25% |
| Low carb | 20% | 50% | 30% |
| High protein/ moderate carb | 40% | 25% | 35% |
| Keto diet | 5% | 75% | 20% |

**Table 15.9** Percentages of calories derived from carbohydrate, protein, and fat in different diets.

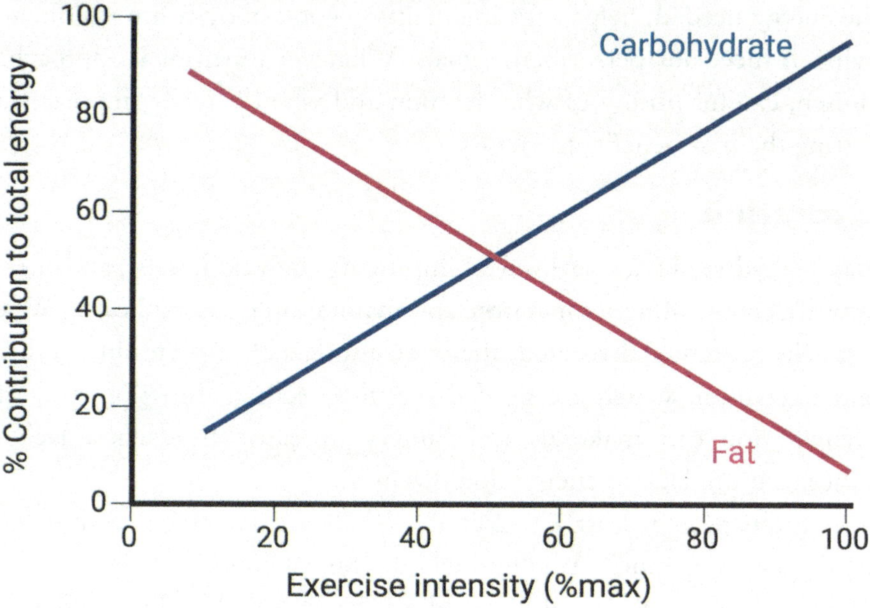


**Figure 15.5** Contribution of carbohydrate and fat to energy supply at different exercise intensities.

instead of carbs, which is not a bad thing unless you have low body fat. But fat sometimes can't be metabolised quickly enough and so protein may be broken down, which also happens if the person has low body fat.

Low carbohydrate diets have not been shown to be effective in assisting muscle recovery and increasing muscle mass in strength and power-based training and in HIIT. Carbohydrates aid muscle recovery, improve neural activity (nerve activation of muscles), and reduce muscle breakdown. So at least moderate carbohydrates are more suitable for strength and power-orientated training.

For those who want to try a lower carb and higher protein diet, the suggestion is to slowly reduce carbs and increase protein in increments to avoid changing too much too soon. With this approach, a balance can be reached that best suits the individual.

How to make sense of all of this? To some extent, the balance of carbs versus protein versus fat is a highly individual thing. For most though, the suggestion is to cut back on carbs, prioritising those with low GI and GL, but beyond that we can experiment with what suits best, gives the energy needed, helps with maintaining good body composition, and helps to meet our performance goals. Whatever nutritional approach is chosen, careful timing of what is eaten and when is really important in getting the best benefits to vitality.

## Hydration

Staying hydrated is a smart way of improving cognition, sleep, and energy as well as controlling temperature and maintaining general health. When our cells become dehydrated, there are also less electrolytes like sodium and potassium, which are needed for those cells to function properly. Dehydration can make us feel hungry or cause headaches, lack of concentration, lack of energy, and dizziness.

Adults need at least 1.5–2 litres of fluid per day, that's around eight to ten glasses or mugs. Any fluid will do, but of course we need to avoid drinks that are high in calories and additives. Suitable fluids are water, coffee or tea, and fruit-flavoured drinks. Up to 30% of our water can come from foods (fruits and vegetables). The suggestion that caffeine doesn't count in hydration is a myth; it has a mild diuretic effect that is easily counteracted by the fluid taken in.

## The When of Nutrition: Timing (Chrono-nutrition)

Our biological clocks have important effects on our energy balance and metabolism, and so we are back to chronobiology, or in this case '**chrono-nutrition**'. As detailed earlier, our circadian rhythms mean that most of us are more alert and focus on cognitive tasks earlier in the day, whereas early in the afternoon many suffer with decreases in cognitive performance. Identical meals eaten at different times of the day can have different effects on cognition, and research indicates that ingested calories are apparently utilised more efficiently in the morning than in the evening and there is better weight control in those who eat earlier. Nevertheless, the eating habits of many are out of synchrony with these biological truths. Gradually increasing energy intake through the day and high evening energy intakes is common across the Western world, with 33–40% of total daily energy intake occurring in the evening in some countries, with the highest being the UK,[229] truly clashing with our innate chronobiology.

As the controller of our twenty-four hour circadian rhythm, the master clock in the hypothalamus of the brain coordinates the peripheral clocks throughout the body, including in the gut, muscles, and all other organs. This is largely influenced by the presence or absence of light. These clocks control timings of eating behaviours, and they also control appetite, digestion, nutrient uptake, and metabolism – all under the higher control of the master clock. We are programmed such that the light cycle stimulates wakefulness and feeding and the dark cycle stimulates sleeping and fasting. When this is disrupted there is the potential for dysregulation of the clocks that control digestion and metabolism and inducement of a pro-inflammatory state that has a negative impact on health and performance.[230]

The timing of food intake and exercise can also influence the clocks (see figure 15.6, *overleaf*). Eating late at night may disrupt the circadian rhythm. Exercising in daylight can help our clocks, particularly in recovering from jet lag.

While a calorie is indeed a calorie, the timing of intake appears to have an impact on how that calorie is metabolised. Night shift workers are known to be more prone to obesity and metabolic disorders, and this has been suggested to relate to circadian rhythm misalignment, independent of energy balance. An increased risk of obesity and related health conditions has been associated with breakfast skipping and late-night feeding and has been associated with circadian disruption. Morning

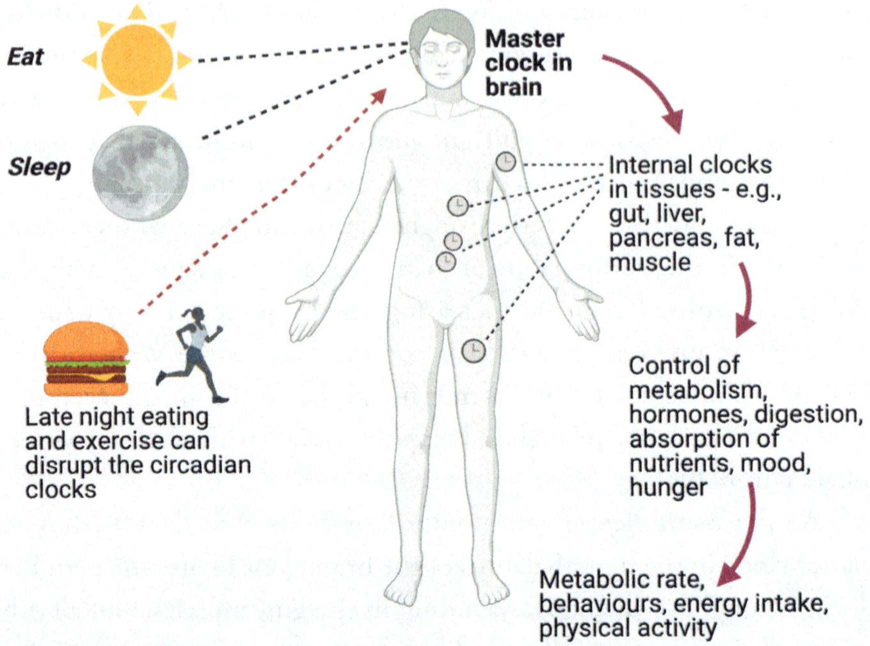


**Figure 15.6** Circadian clocks and their effects.

energy intake may have substantial health benefits, and evening energy consumption has been associated with higher BMI. The collective research indicates that the later calories are consumed, the less benefit they have.[231]

One study divided ninety-three overweight women into two groups; one group mostly having morning calorie consumption (50% calories at breakfast and 14% at dinner) and one group having evening consumption (14% calories at breakfast and 50% at dinner). The morning consumption group resulted in a 5.1 kg greater weight loss relative to the evening calorie consumption group, and the difference was significant by the fourth week.[232] The reasons may relate to different behaviours due to the change in eating habits and/or the difference of circadian rhythms on the metabolism of food.

Breakfast seems to have a higher impact on cognitive performance than does lunch, and there is some evidence that indicates that consumption of lunch may impair cognitive performance and negatively alter mood. A drop in performance of mental tasks and a decline in mood are seen an hour after consuming lunch and may take several hours to return to a pre-lunch state, but this may partly relate to the fact that our chronobiology means that we are less alert in the afternoon anyway.[233] Nevertheless, the declines seem greater in those who have consumed lunch, meaning that food intake really does contribute to the 'post-lunch dip', especially if the lunch is big. It is reasonable to suggest that, given high carbohydrate meals can result in increased drowsiness, lunch should be protein-orientated and small in size. Notably, evidence suggests that consumption of an afternoon snack (e.g., an 250 ml yoghurt) may help to alleviate some of the performance decrements seen in the afternoon.

There is less research on the effects of the evening meal specifically on cognitive performance, probably because people tend to do less cognitively demanding tasks in the evening. Those who have evening meals show better logical reasoning skills and are subjectively stronger and more motivated than those who do not.[234]

## Fasting and Time-Restricted Eating

The new interest in 'chrono-nutrition' has merged to some extent with that of fasting. There is no doubt that fasting improves insulin sensitivity, and intermittent fasting such as the 5:2 diet or variations on that theme are effective in improving many aspects of cardiometabolic health, inflammation and oxidative stress, fat accumulation, and assisting weight loss.[235] These are diets where the calories are restricted – for example to 800 kcal a day for a woman or 900 for a man – for a few days per week, and 'normal' eating happens on the other days. The expectation is that a 'new normal' develops that is healthier, as opposed to being able to overeat on the non-fasting days and expecting it to work. Stores of glycogen (stored glucose) begin to run low around ten to twelve hours after their last meal, and at that stage it is expected that the body switches into fat-burning mode and uses ketones instead of glucose. That switch is often associated with initial hunger, fatigue, and headaches, which continue for a few days if the fasting continues and then fades away.

Another 'mini-fasting' approach is to follow a time-restricted eating pattern, which more reflects the suggestions from chrono-nutrition. Eat only during specific hours of the day, for example twelve hours, or even more extreme, eight hours; don't eat or drink anything with calories outside of that window; and eat at set mealtimes in that window only. Proposed benefits of time restricted eating include increased insulin sensitivity, improved metabolism, lower blood pressure, and a lower appetite in the evening. Less radical than other fasting approaches, it is often more acceptable and easier to maintain as a life-long habit. It really is more about regimenting one's schedule; yet again, timing is everything.[236]

## How to Improve Insulin Sensitivity

It is clear that improving insulin sensitivity is a smart way of improving performance; it can improve health and well-being, sleep quality, appetite, and body composition. The basic steps to achieve this are:

- Regular exercise has a powerful influence on insulin sensitivity.
- Choose what to eat: aim for low GI and GL foods.
- Keep overall carbohydrate load under control.
- Optimise good protein, don't avoid good fat.
- Choose when to eat: Timing is everything. Consider time-restricted eating.
- Stay hydrated: drink plenty of water throughout the day

If you are interested in understanding how to use nutrition to optimise performance in sport and to recover after exercise training, the next chapter will provide insights. Further approaches to reducing body fat while maintaining an exercise regime are included there.

**Key Messages:**

- Nutrition influences vitality and performance through its widespread effects on the brain and peripheral organs, influencing many aspects of mental function, metabolism, fitness, and health.
- The brain-gut index plays a major role in our responses to nutrition. The gut microbiome is negatively affected by bad diets and some medicines.
- Insulin sensitivity is central to considering best nutrition strategies, and part of enhancing sensitivity is to reduce carbs intake and focus on low GL, optimise protein, and plan eating times according to our circadian rhythms.
- High sugar intake is an addiction and is linked to poor cognition, significant negative physical and mental health effects, and inevitably reduced performance.
- How we metabolise food is influenced by our body clocks: timing is important to get best effects.
- The Mediterranean diet is a good template upon which to build an individualised nutrition programme.

## The Truth about Supplements

The world of supplementation and 'nutraceuticals' is very big business and full of hype. Most of these supplements are a waste of time, they will not make a bad diet good, and they may cause harm. Many who take supplements exceed the recommended dose, which can be toxic. Many sports supplements are not what they seem; they can contain things not stated on the packaging and/or be missing the things they claim to provide! This underpins the reason why supplements that elite athletes take have to be 'batch tested' to ensure they are what they say they are and do not contain substances that are banned.

There is an additional issue relating to supplements that is very important to health and performance, and that is the fact that nutrients in foods interact with one another to make them not only better absorbed but also more effective in the body. Gaining nutrients from a healthy diet must always be the first approach.

What supplements are worth discussing? First we will discuss those for general health and then supplements used by athletes.

## Supplements for General Health

**Vitamin D**, the sunshine vitamin is a hormone that is essential for muscle and bone health, and it is considered to support the immune system and confer other health benefits. The most convincing effects are on the musculoskeletal system. Vitamin D is converted by sunshine from a precursor in the skin to its active component, D3, and therefore sun exposure is needed to have optimal levels. The problem with that is that it increases the risk of melanoma, and also the farther away from the equator people live, the more months of the year they will not have adequate exposure to direct sunshine. Furthermore, if you have darker skin, your levels are often lower. It is no surprise then that a large portion of the world's population is vitamin D deficient, and so most will benefit from a supplement, even 1,000 International Units (IU) of vitamin D3 daily, taken after food with some fat in it (e.g., your main meal) to aid absorption.

**Calcium** is very important for general health, particularly bone health. You need about 1,000–1,200 mg/day. Supplements are widely taken, but often unnecessarily so. The body absorbs calcium much better if it is obtained in the diet, for example from dairy products, milk substitutes like almond milk, fatty fish, pulses, seeds, dark green leafy vegetables, or fortified flour products. Taking excessive supplements of calcium has been linked to heart disease. If you want to assess how much calcium you are getting in your diet, try the International Osteoporosis Foundation's calcium calculator at https://www.iofbonehealth.org/calcium-calculator.

**Iron** is an essential element in our diets, attained form a variety of sources. It helps to prevent anaemia, where there are not enough red blood cells to carry oxygen to your tissues. Women are commonly iron deficient, as are those with poor diets, and athletes are also more likely to be iron deficient. Iron deficiency causes fatigue and can reduce physical and mental performance. It is also linked to sleep disruption, restless legs, irritability, and headaches. Hence, iron levels should be checked in those who are fatigued; even a slightly low level can be enough to cause fatigue. In those found to be iron deficient, the cause must be identified, nutritional habits reviewed, and daily supplementation is usually recommended at least short term. People who are prone to iron deficiency (e.g., menstruating women and athletes who train hard) may benefit from intermittent supplementation long term. Some find that difficult to tolerate in the gut, but intermittent supplementation (a few times a week) can be as effective as daily. Note, however, that it is dangerous to over-supplement with iron.

Iron can and should be obtained from a whole range of sources in the diet. There are two forms of dietary iron: heme and non-heme. Heme iron is derived from haemoglobin. It is found in animal foods that originally contained haemoglobin, such as red meats, fish, and poultry (which contain both heme and non-heme iron). Your body absorbs the most iron from heme sources.

Most non-heme iron is from plant sources such as lentils, beans, tofu, spinach, and fortified cereals. Some breads, nuts, and seeds have non-heme iron. This is also the form of iron added to iron-enriched and iron-fortified foods. Our bodies are less efficient at absorbing non-heme iron, but most dietary iron is non-heme iron.

**Vitamin C** plays a number of roles in different systems of the body. It is essential for tissue development as well as healing and repair, and it plays a role in the immune system. It can help iron absorption, and so drinking a glass of orange juice during a meal with good iron content is smart. The recommended daily dietary intake varies between countries but is typically 75–90 mg per day for adults.[237] Much is made of the role of vitamin C in reducing the incidence of the common cold and shortening the duration of an illness, but the evidence suggests this is not the case in the general population. However, in those who regularly exercise intensively, supplementation may help in this respect, and a supplement of less than 1,000 mg daily is generally considered safe.[238]

**Fish oils** are those that contain the unsaturated omega-3 fatty acids EPA and DHA. Products differ in how much of each they have. Dietary intake of these is usually below 200 mg/day, but 500 mg/day should be the target. Sources include fatty fish like salmon, mackerel, and sardines. Some plants – for example flaxseeds, chia seeds, pumpkin seeds, walnuts, and canola oil – are rich in another type of omega-3 fatty acid: alpha-linolenic acid, which the body converts to DHA and EPA.

Fish oil supplements are one of the most common supplements taken globally, as they improve heart and brain health and protect against inflammation and cancers. The evidence in fact is mixed, and overall it isn't convincing, but they may be helpful particularly in those who don't eat any fish. The key message is that it is better to get sources from your diet.

**Probiotics** are live organisms that confer health benefits when consumed in adequate amounts. They are one of the most commonly used supplements and are found as additives to foods such as yoghurt, cheese, breakfast cereals, and various snacks. The rationale for their use has been highlighted in relation to the gut microbiome described earlier, but the evidence for their benefits is mixed, partly because it is likely some micro-organism strains may be more beneficial than others, the potential uses vary, and the quality of research can be poor. As yet, though promising, their routine use in a healthy population is not yet recommended. They are often proposed to be taken after a course of antibiotics or gastrointestinal infection to repopulate the gut with 'healthy' flora. Products vary; yet again, beware of duds.[239]

**Curcumin** is a molecule derived from **turmeric**. It has protective effects on health through antioxidant and anti-inflammatory mechanisms. It is beneficial in protecting against metabolic diseases such as diabetes, cardiovascular and neurological diseases, cancer, and arthritis. The doses needed have not been determined, and so it is logical simply to add the spice to meals where appropriate.[240]

## Supplements in Sport

**Protein** supplements for recovery (in powder form) can be more acceptable to many individuals and, providing they are not tainted with hidden products, are sensible. Similarly, some people like liquid meal supplements: carbohydrate rich, moderate protein, low fat powders with some vitamins. Again, these are okay as long as they fit into the overall nutrition plan.

**Caffeine** assists with performance in events lasting more than one minute, showing benefits in performance in short duration super maximal exercise (one to five minutes), sustained high intensity exercise (twenty to sixty minutes), and endurance exercise of more than sixty minutes. Caffeine raises alertness, enhances the sense of energy, and reduces the perception of pain. If ingested about an hour before exercise, it can enhance muscle strength, endurance, and performance in high intensity exercise. Perceived exertion is lower with caffeine on board, and it can improve reaction times and motor coordination. This is true for both habitual and non-habitual coffee drinkers. An average cup of instant coffee contains 50–70 mg, filtered coffee has 60–120 mg, and tea has 10–50 mg, and there are plenty of other beverages that include caffeine. Even 1.5 mg/kg, forty-five to sixty minutes before a session can be effective. Caffeine can also increase basal metabolic rate (your energy expenditure at rest) although not by much. The evidence for this is mixed, and some people respond, while some don't. Note also that caffeine toxicity can occur, which results in a range of effects such as palpitations and anxiety and more serious consequences. This has sadly become more common with the advent of energy gels with high caffeine content.

**Creatine** supplementation (creatine monohydrate) has been a popular choice among strength and sprint/power athletes. But the gains may be extremely small if there already is a smart nutritional strategy and a well-designed training programme in place. Nevertheless, given its popularity and its effectiveness in those who are not reaching protein requirements otherwise, it is discussed here. Creatine allows greater load to be maintained in strength training, and increases strength, power, and muscle mass. It has no benefits in endurance events. It can be unsafe in those with any risk factors for kidney problems, and also beware of tainted supplements. There are two regimes: (1) a loading dose of 20 g/day for four to five days, then maintenance dose of 2–3 g/day; or (2) a maintenance dose of 2–3 g/day for thirty days. Some recommend taking 50–100 g carbohydrate to enhance loading. Exercise also enhances uptake into the muscle. Once the loading has been achieved, the creatine will take about four weeks to return to resting levels, unless maintenance with 2–3 g/day is continued.[241]

Supplementation with **beta-alanine** and **sodium bicarbonate** (300 mg/kg, ninety minutes before the event, though some spread the dose over two to three hours) may lead to a small improvement in performance in events lasting forty seconds to ten minutes. **Sodium citrate** can have the same effects. One to two litres of water should be taken in at the same time, with some carbohydrate. A lot of people find bicarb and citrate cause gastrointestinal upset.

**Probiotics** may be more useful in athletes who are travelling and training intensively, as there is a higher incidence of gastrointestinal disturbance and changes in gut function, in addition to other issues such as upper respiratory tract infections. It has been recommended that they be considered in this group to aid nutrient absorption, provide immune support, and assist recovery from intensive exercise.[242]

# 16

# Nutrition for Exercise and Recovery

## Guidance for More Serious Athletes

This chapter provides an overview of elements of nutrition that apply to those who are more serious about their fitness training, and this simply means anyone following a formal programme involving regular exercise sessions most days of the week. Eating and drinking to recover is key to making a programme successful and to performing well. *Timing is critical*, and fuel intake after exercise will depend on the aims – short-term recovery to exercise again soon, or long-term recovery if there is a longer interval between exercise bouts (eight to twenty-four hours).[243]

**Hydration** is always vital, and we need to add further fluid intake with exercise and even more so if we are in hot climates. The suggestion is to start the session hydrated; drink 400–600 ml fluid two hours before exercise, and if it is a long endurance event, drink 300–500 ml, fifteen minutes beforehand if possible. For exercise that lasts over an hour, the aim is to drink 150–250 ml every fifteen minutes; drinking smaller volumes more often may be easier on the stomach.

It is not common, but it is possible to overhydrate if the amounts taken in are significantly higher than described, or in the scenario of running at a very slow pace, when drinking these amounts every fifteen minutes may result in too much fluid being taken on board, which reduces sodium levels (hyponatraemia), and that's dangerous. The symptoms are headaches, nausea, vomiting, and confusion. Urine colour is a very good indicator of hydration status: pale yellow urine suggests good fluid balance, darker urine means dehydration, and colourless means overhydration. If body weight before the session/event is the same afterwards, then that indicates good fluid balance. For every kg lost in fluid, it takes about 1.2–1.5 litres to compensate.

## Food and Recovery

Nutritional strategies to recover after exercise actually start *before* we exercise, and indeed they start with the recovery strategy after the previous session. Starting to exercise with low glycogen stores in our muscles causes inferior performance and greater fatigue. *You can't pour from an empty cup.*

Eating small amounts of protein, carbohydrate, and perhaps leucine (a valuable amino acid) shortly before, during, and after intensive exercise may help with muscle recovery. Also, eating soon after an exercise session helps to restore muscle glycogen and to repair and remodel muscle. Eating as early as possible takes advantage of the enhanced rate of muscle glycogen storage, especially in the first hour post-exercise, which helps us to be ready for the next session. Immediate intake is particularly important for those exercising again within eight hours; so for short-term recovery, early intake is key.[244]

For those training again within eight hours, the recommendation for carbohydrate is to take in 1–1.2 g of carbohydrate per kg body weight every hour for four hours after exercise, or the equivalent amount eaten in a single meal or series of snacks in that time period.

The timing isn't so critical if one is not exercising again within twenty-four hours, although starting to replenish within two hours is best. Consuming adequate daily carbohydrate (independent of its pattern and/or timing) is the most important nutritional strategy to maximize muscle glycogen resynthesis with prolonged (i.e., >8 hours) post-exercise recovery. If high volume training for three days in a row is performed, muscle glycogen will decline even on a moderately high (5–7 g/kg/day) diet. Consuming a carbohydrate-rich diet (i.e., approximately 12 g/kg/day) as two large meals as compared with seven smaller meals results in similar net muscle glycogen synthesis over twenty-four hours.

The type of carbohydrate consumed in recovery can also be important. It seems more effective if high glycaemic index carbs are ingested for the first few hours after exercise, so the carbs get to the muscles and restore glycogen, and then low glycaemic carbs are consumed for the rest of the day to control hunger and keep insulin levels stable.

## What about Protein?

The consensus now is that replenishing both protein and carbohydrate is important.[245] Since protein also supports repair and remodelling of muscle, it is important in recovery nutrition. Protein alone won't work to resynthesize glycogen, but if carbohydrate is suboptimal (1 g/kg/hour or less), then adding protein can also particularly help glycogen resynthesis. What we eat to recover depends on the exercise we have done, of course. More research has been done on protein intake after strength-based work than after endurance exercise.

Ingesting protein + carb soon after training reduces the cortisol level seen during and after exercise. Since cortisol, a stress hormone, causes muscle breakdown, it is beneficial to reduce it in this context. So in summary: combined carb and protein ingestion soon after exercise will result in benefit through (a) replenishing muscle glycogen stores quickly, (b) reduction in cortisol, hence reducing muscle breakdown, and (c) stimulate muscle repair.

In nutrition specifically for recovery, protein type is important in any recovery snack. Casein (from milk) causes a moderate and prolonged increase in protein availability, whereas whey (also from milk) results in more rapid but shorter responses. Chocolate milk is an excellent recovery drink; it has carbohydrate, electrolytes, and fluids and has milk (casein and whey) proteins. The whey protein has the advantage of rapid absorption; the casein has the advantage of prolonged release of amino acids. When it comes to post-exercise meals to enhance recovery, fish protein is a good choice as it has a positive effect on insulin sensitivity and all the amino acids needed. Vegetable proteins seem less effective, possibly due to difference in digestion and lower amino acids scores. Also, vegan diets are associated with higher cortisol levels, which can cause muscle breakdown rather than recovery.

- **250–350 ml milkshake or chocolate milk**
- **250 ml fat-free yoghurt or 350 ml low-fat drinking yoghurt**
- **Sandwich with lean protein filling (e.g., chicken, egg) + 1 piece of fruit**
- **1 high protein bar (beware fat) > 10 g protein + glass of fruit juice**
- **250–350 ml fruit smoothie (fruit, low fat yoghurt, honey)**
- **250–350 ml carb drink + 250 ml liquid meal supplement with >10 g protein**

**Table 16.1** Examples of healthy recovery snacks.

## Carb Loading before an Event and Requirements for Endurance/Ultra-Endurance Training

Carbohydrate loading in advance of endurance events (e.g., a marathon) has long been used as a performance nutrition strategy and can be very useful, although it does not suit everyone. This is where a high carb diet is followed for the three days before the event (7–10 g/kg/day) to ensure the muscles are fully replenished with glycogen. This can be reduced to twenty-four to thirty-six hours prior to the event if the 10 g/kg level is adhered to.

Some endurance athletes advocate the 'train low, compete high' approach, whereby they train at least part of their time in a fasted state (early morning sessions), but carb load before an event. The proposed advantage of training in a fasted state is that it encourages metabolic adaptation to using fat as a fuel, but it has mixed effects.

Nutritional requirements for endurance training are described in table 16.2. Individuals are encouraged to evaluate different carbohydrate intakes across the ranges given to assess their impact on their performance and recovery.

| Goal | Suggested carb intake |
|---|---|
| **Daily intake to fuel light activity or exercise <60–90 MVPA* minutes/day** | 5–7 g/kg[+]/day |
| **Daily intake for those training >90–120 MVPA* minutes/day** | 7–10 g/kg/day** |
| **During exercise: carb intake during sessions >60–90 minutes** | 45–60 g/hour<br>Eg., 300–400 ml carb drink + 1 banana; or 4–5 jelly beans + large banana |
| **Post exercise: to promote recovery, especially when exercising again within 8 hours** | 1–1.2 g/kg/hour in first few hours |

[+] g/kg means grams of carb per kg body weight.

***** Moderate to Vigorous Physical Activity.

****** Those who wish to carb load for longer events may aim for the higher end of this range.

Note the usual recommendations still apply: high GI carbs post-exercise and lower GI carbs in the rest of the day.

**Table 16.2** Carbohydrate intake for specific training purposes.

Here are some examples of a pre-endurance exercise meal/snack, three to four hours before a session (200–300 g carb):

- Porridge + low fat milk or yoghurt
- 2 slices toast + scrambled egg and glass of fruit juice
- Low fat/fibre sports bar + cup of fruit juice/energy drink

Endurance athletes need more protein than sedentary people, but evidence on the exact amount needed for best performance is limited, and it probably depends on the individual.[246] Typically, though, 1.2–1.7 g/kg of protein are recommended. This can usually be met with a healthy balanced diet. There seems to be no benefits to going above this level as an endurance athlete.

Some of this protein should be taken in during the early recovery period after exercise. Here are some examples of 10 g protein:

- 40–50 g lean meat, chicken, fish, low fat cheese, or nuts (watch out for fat content though)
- 2 eggs
- 300 ml skim milk
- ½– ¾ cup dried beans, lentils, or split peas

## Nutritional Requirements for Strength/Resistance Training

Strength training promotes muscle mass providing there is proper nutrition. Eating – and in particular, protein intake – is vital to achieving a good response to resistance training. Resistance training makes a muscle 'anabolically sensitive' to protein intake such that it builds in this time window.[247]

Ingesting 20–25g protein or 10g amino acids, results in maximum stimulation of muscle protein synthesis. Protein intake greater than 25g has limited positive effects on muscle. As described earlier, whey protein is the rapid protein component of milk and is high in leucine; it results in maximum increases in muscle response when taken early after training. Ingesting protein before or during a resistance session has not been convincingly demonstrated to be effective. Carbohydrate, while important to restore muscle glycogen, doesn't have an impact on muscle protein synthesis. Note though that one bout of resistance training can deplete muscle glycogen by 25–40%, and this needs replenishing with carbs or performance will drop.

Advice for gaining the best effects of resistance training is therefore as follows: consume protein as soon as possible after training. For lighter athletes, less than 20 g is needed. For bigger (>85 kg) athletes, 20–25 g of high quality protein is best. Whey protein seems best for this purpose. Adding some carbohydrate to the protein after resistance work helps to restore the glycogen so that the energy stores are there, but this does not build muscle. There is no advantage to exceeding 1.6–1.7 g/protein/kg/day, and indeed, consuming more than this can be detrimental.

What about sprint events, where power to weight ratio is important? Similar principles apply to those with resistance training: a high protein diet may confer an advantage. Carbohydrate is important for muscle energy stores and performance, but 3–7 g/kg/day is adequate for those who train one to two hours daily.

Middle distance athletes need to be primed for both speed and endurance. This group have the most varied training programmes, so the nutrition plan is also quite varied. However carbohydrate intake should be around 7–10 g/kg/day (55–70% or more of the total energy intake), recovery enhanced by intake of 1.2–1.5 g/kg/hour carbs and 0.3 g/kg/hour for the first few hours after training. Fat should be reduced to about 20% of total intake.

## Lowering Body Fat

It is news to no one that a balanced diet, regular exercise, and careful planning of what we eat and when are the keys to weight management. If the aim is to lose body fat, then sensible weight loss goals are around 0.5–1 kg per week, no more. That's a reduction of about 5 mm in total skinfolds per week, and it is around 500–1,000 kcal per day less calories. For females, energy intake should not drop below 30–35 kcal/kg of fat free mass per day, because less than that can cause serious hormonal abnormalities that affect many aspects of health.

Carbohydrate intake at 3–5 g/kg for those doing light and moderate exercise is recommended. This can increase to 6–8 g/kg in those who engage in strenuous exercise. Carbohydrates should be those that are rich in nutrients (fruit, vegetables, pasta, porridges, wholegrains) rather than carb drinks, bars, or sweets. Protein should be 1.4–1.7 g/kg (upper end of the limit if there is serious calorie restriction), and fat should be kept to 1–1.5 g/kg/day and <30% of the energy intake. There should not be reduction of fat intake below 15% of total energy intake because it will impair the immune system

Avoiding calories for ninety minutes after exercise will optimise fat burning. The problem is that this will significantly reduce post-exercise recovery, meaning that the ability to exercise the next time will be reduced, so it doesn't work well.

| |
|---|
| **Planning**<br>• Plan eating schedules for the day/week, including to assist recovery after exercise. Allow a 'metabolic window' of at least twelve hours fasting.<br>• Stick to low GI carbs except soon after exercise.<br>• Don't skimp on protein.<br>• If possible, time the exercise sessions to before a meal.<br>• If you are sedentary or only doing light activity, don't eat like an athlete! |
| **Avoid empty calories**<br>• Stay hydrated; drink water regularly; avoid calorie-laden drinks.<br>• Minimise snacking. |
| **Watch out for unnecessary fats**<br>• Choose lean protein, watch out for 'health/sport/energy' bars that have high fat content, often saturated fat.<br>• Beware fat- and calorie-containing sauces.<br>• Avoid fried food and foods grilled in butter/oil.<br>• Choose healthy snacks without fat (e.g., fruit, vegetables). |

**Table 16.3** Tips to achieving lower body fat.

## Overdoing It: Low Energy Availability

**Energy in – energy out = Energy availability**. There are some who, in the drive to get fitter, lose weight, have the 'perfect body', or for deeper psychological reasons, get the energy balance challenge wrong in the opposite direction to those who overeat. Low energy intake compared to needs results in low energy availability, and although this may be part of a weight loss programme, it can go too far. Energy availability <30 kcal/

fat free mass per day is dangerous to health. It threatens bones, causes muscle loss, changes your metabolic rate in a downward direction, and harms sexual and reproductive health. Relative energy deficiency in sport (REDS) is a common problem now, in both genders, and is a form of eating disorder. Don't go there.[248]

**Key Messages:**

- The timing of energy intake during and after exercise has a major impact on performance, metabolism, and recover.
- Both protein and carbohydrate are essential for recovery.
- Carbohydrate levels should be regulated according to the type and intensity of training.
- Carbohydrate loading can benefit those in endurance events.
- The balance of carbohydrate and protein intake and its timing in relation to training can be highly individual; one size does not fit all.
- Beware low energy balance.

# 17

# Sleep to Succeed

## Sleep Well, Perform Better

*Next time you see someone sleeping, make believe you're in a science fiction movie, and whisper, 'The creature is regenerating itself.'*

**George Carlin**

### Why Is Sleep So Important?

As a physician and scientist, I always find it extraordinary that people will make huge efforts to get fit and eat well, and then completely ignore their night-time health. Sleep restores us. It is special and personal and is a vital element of our holistic health, well-being, and performance. While sleeping, our bodies recover, cells repair, tissues are restored, and our brains partly rest and partly stay very active, attending to 'housework', continuing to control hormones and metabolism, and processing information from the day and storing some of it in memory. If sleep has been adequate, we wake physically and mentally refreshed and ready for the day ahead.

On average, we spend a third of our time sleeping (or we should do), and as is increasingly recognised, if we don't have good sleep, many negative consequences can follow. Some of those are obvious: poor performance, low energy, brain fog, greater hunger, lower mood. Unfortunately, that's the tip of the iceberg: those with poor sleep habits are at much higher risk of a whole range of diseases.[249] The impact of insufficient sleep is enormous, both on the individual and on society. Insufficient sleep increases mortality by up to 13% and is linked to seven of the fifteen leading causes of death: cardiovascular disease, cancer, cerebrovascular disease, accidents, diabetes, septicaemia, and hypertension.[250] Adults who are short sleepers are statistically significantly more likely to be obese and physically inactive, and are more likely to be smokers. After four nights of sleep restriction, insulin sensitivity decreases by a massive 29%![251] No surprises then that poor sleep makes it harder to lose weight, as well as making it harder to get fit, and harder to perform at work and to feel good about life. Many of the associations between sleep, health, and performance are bidirectional – for example, if we have pain we sleep less well, and if we sleep less well our pain is worse.

Sleep loss has a major impact on performance, impairing health and well-being, cognitive performance, overall performance at work, and productivity. Lack of sleep leads to more accidents and has been linked to a range of disasters such as the Chernobyl nuclear explosion, the Three Mile Island nuclear incident, the Exxon Valdez spill, and the Space Shuttle Challenger tragedy.[252] Friendly fire deaths in the military have also been attributed to sleep deprivation.

| | |
|---|---|
| **Brain** | 33% ↑ risk of dementia<br>58% ↑ risk of depression, other mood disorders<br>The brain ages by 3–5 years<br>Significant cognitive impairment, brain fog, memory lapses |
| **Metabolism** | 50% ↑ risk of obesity with <5 hours/night<br>3x more likely to get diabetes |
| **Heart and circulation** | 48% ↑ risk of heart disease, strokes<br>↑ risk high blood pressure |
| **Cancer** | ↑ risk of cancer |
| **Other organs** | >40% risk lung diseases<br>30% ↑ risk of kidney disease |
| **Immune system** | 3x more likely to catch colds, viruses, and higher risk of other infections |
| **Accidents and injuries** | ↑ risk of accidents and injuries<br>↑ risk of poor healing after injury<br>Poor recovery after exercise |

**Table 17.1** Some consequences of insufficient sleep.

| Country | Percentage sleeping < 7 hours/ night | Total days lost due to insufficient sleep | Total hours lost due to insufficient sleep | Annual loss of GDP |
|---|---|---|---|---|
| **USA** | 45% | 1,234,864 | 9,878,910 | $411 billion (2.28%) |
| **UK** | 35% | 207,224 | 1,657,792 | $50 billion (1.86%) |
| **Germany** | 30% | 209,024 | 1,672,192 | $60 billion (1.56%) |
| **Japan** | 56% | 604,191 | 5,833,532 | $138 billion (2.92%) |
| **Canada** | 26% | 78,861 | 630,886 | $21.4 billion (1.35%) |

**Table 17.2** Loss of productivity due to sleep loss across 5 OECD countries.[253]

## Sleep Homeostasis: Balancing Sleep and Wakefulness

Sleep is defined as: '*a reversible behavioural state of perceptual disengagement from, and unresponsiveness to, the environment*'.[254] When we are awake and when we are asleep is largely controlled by our internal clocks that control our circadian rhythms and our sleep drive, and this whole balancing act is called '**sleep homeostasis**'.[xi] These two mechanisms regulate brain activity and the balance of different chemicals that either promote alertness or sleep. Through these processes, our circadian rhythms promote wakefulness by supporting signals to keep us alert in the day, acting in opposition to our '**sleep drive**', which supports our biological need for sleep. This sleep drive is always switched on, but at some times of the day it is at a low setting – particularly after we have had a good night's sleep. In good circumstances, our internal clocks make us awake and alert for around sixteen hours, and our internal clock 'alert' signals oppose the

xi. Homeostasis: the process of maintaining a stable internal environment suitable for sustaining life.

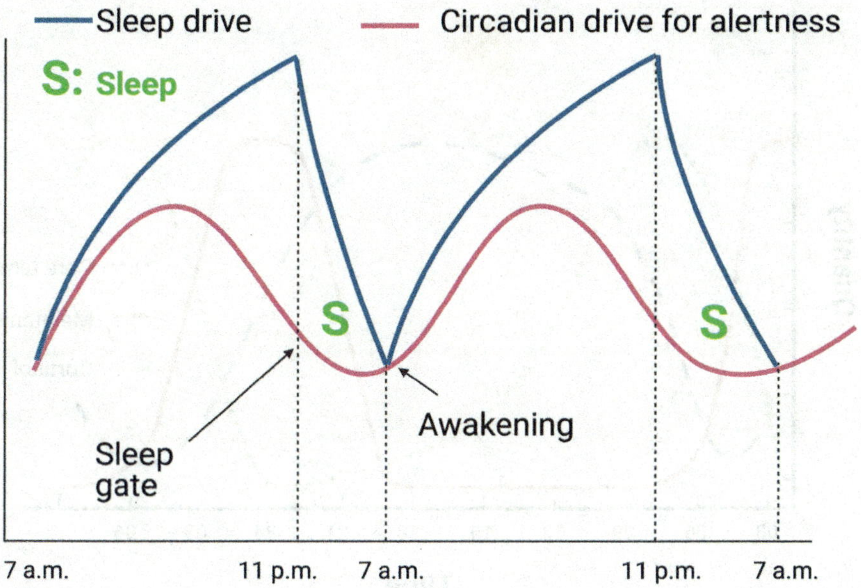


**Figure 17.1** The sleep homeostat.

increasing sleep drive that occurs during the day. Then the alert signals decline, the sleep drive becomes dominant, and we are ready for sleep. In the first half of the night our sleep drive remains dominant, but after around four hours it starts to decline, and our internal clocks starts to work in different ways to support ongoing sleep.[255]

There are many chemicals (neurotransmitters) that influence the sleep-wake cycle, and also many hormones fluctuate as part of the same process, but the hormone that largely helps to regulate sleep is melatonin. You will recall from chapter 12 (Chronobiology) that this is released by the pineal gland in the mid-brain. Levels are high in darkness, and the level starts to rise as dusk falls; this period is called the sleep gate, and we will sleep best if we go to sleep during this time (see figure 17.2). When daylight arrives, melatonin levels fall, and this is why natural light (or a daylight lamp in the winter) is important for natural waking.

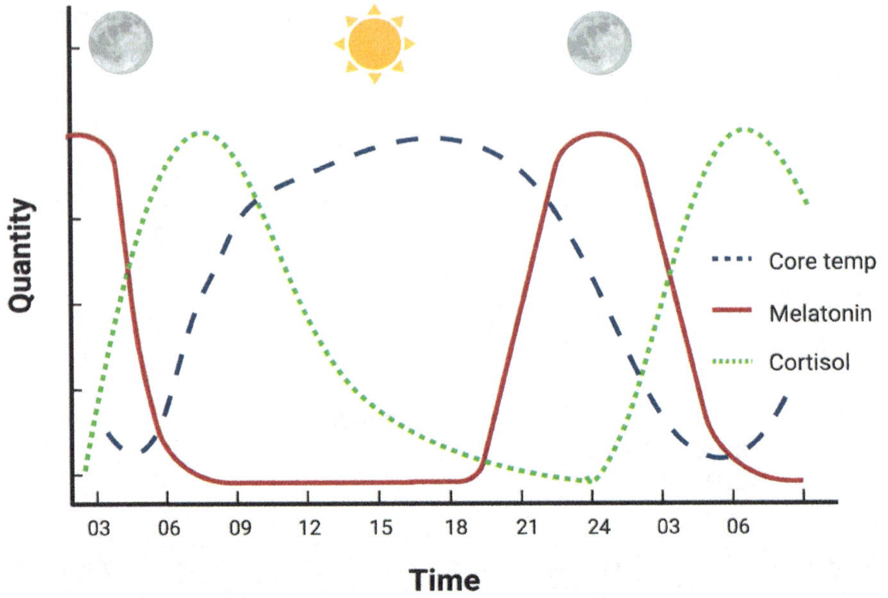


**Figure 17.2** Melatonin, cortisol, and core body temperature changes across the 24-hour sleep-wake cycle.

## Clearly Sleep Is Important, but How Does It Work?

Sleep science is complex, and frankly, we still don't understand the meaning of many elements of sleep. When the authors of a major textbook on sleep state, '*The function of sleep remains the greatest biologic mystery of all times*',[256] it is not surprising that the rest of us find it an intimidating thing to figure out. Many will get bogged down by the science and metrics that are frequently involved in any information about sleep. Health technologies offer a whole range of metrics that, while helpful in some ways and holding promise for the future, can leave the user confused as to what they mean and how to use them. The best approach is to focus on those elements where there is greatest understanding and that are relevant to vitality and performance.

### What Is Good Sleep?

Good sleep means good quality and good quantity. Most adults need seven to nine hours sleep (that's 'sleep need'). There are few who perform well on less, and most of those who think they can are, in fact, chronically sleep deprived. Albert Einstein reportedly slept ten hours per night. Serious/professional athletes may need more than nine hours (e.g., LeBron James and Roger Federer are both reported to need twelve hours).

Sleep can be measured according to our perception of sleep quality, the duration of our sleep, how long it takes to get to sleep (latency), and how many times we wake in the night (awakenings). 'Sleep efficiency' means how long we sleep compared to how long we lie in bed. 'Sleep consistency' means how consistent we are in the timing of going to bed and getting up, assessed across days and weeks.

| Dimension | Description |
|---|---|
| **Duration** | Total time spent asleep. Good: 7–9 hours. |
| **Latency** | Amount of time to go to sleep after getting into bed. Ideally less than 20 minutes. |
| **Efficiency** | The percentage time spent asleep while in bed. Good: >85% |
| **Consolidation** | Based on the number of sleep bouts. Bouts are broken by awakenings. You may not notice the number of times you are awake intermittently in the night as these can be very short. Good: not certain, probably <4 bouts of wakening. |
| **Consistency** | Regularity of sleep and waking times. |

**Table 17.3** Important dimensions of sleep.

Sleep goes in cycles throughout the night, from waking, to very light sleep, then the Rapid Eye Movement (REM) phase when we dream, and then shallow non-REM sleep stages N1 and N2, and deep 'slow wave' sleep (non-REM stage N3). There are about five cycles of sleep per night, each lasting around ninety minutes, but this varies across the night and also across individuals.

Our sleep rhythms, their susceptibility to other stimuli, the consequences of changes, and the effectiveness of interventions may be

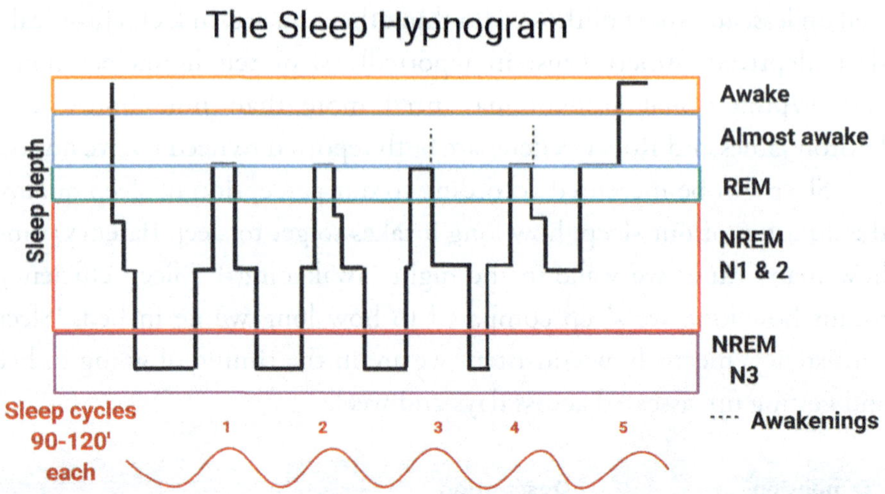


**Figure 17.3** The sleep hypnogram: Each sleep cycle lasts about 90 minutes and consists of different sleep stages.

| Stage | Description |
|---|---|
| **REM** | Dreamy sleep. Starts after the first 90 minutes. Initially short but increases with each cycle in the night. Heart rate and blood pressure slightly increase, breathing quickens and becomes more shallow, and muscles completely relax. The brain is active in this phase, processing information from the day that can then be stored in long-term memory.<br>Typically amounts to 20–25% of total sleep duration. |
| **Non-REM, Stages N1–N2** | Stages N1 and N2 are light sleep. |
| **Non-REM, Stage N3** | Stage N3 is deep, refreshing sleep and typically accounts for 15–20% sleep time, but in some people it is as high as 35%. The amount decreases with age. There is more in the first half of the night than in the second. |
| Stage N2 and REM are the largest share of sleep time (60–85%). | |

**Table 17.4** A description of sleep stages.

highly variable between individuals. The absolute amount of deep non-REM sleep may predict how refreshed we feel in the morning, but the specific functions of other sleep stages are less clear. Imbalanced light sleep versus deep sleep may indicate some sleep disorders; for example, in sleep apnoea deep sleep is lacking. Brief, fragmented sleep has little or no recuperative value and is similar to total sleep deprivation in its effects on performance.

Sleep can be measured in a number of ways, including through 'polysomnography' in a sleep laboratory setting where brain, heart, and sleep activity are recorded, and this is where research and clinical studies may be carried out. For more 'real world' assessment, we can evaluate our sleep status using a simple quality score (scale of 0–10), and we might use a more extensive sleep log,[xii] which is completed every morning for seven days to provide insights into sleep quality and quantity.

Many people also use technologies. There are a range of devices that offer sleep monitoring, including watches, bands, rings, and devices in the room, including our phones. They can offer information on the dimensions and stages of sleep described. They do not replace keeping a personal log and reflecting on sleep quality, and there are many that as yet are not very reliable in relation to sleep staging, but they can still provide valuable information on time spent asleep, awakenings, and latency, and so they may offer useful insights. They also help just by making the user focus on optimising their sleep. Note my usual warning with using these devices: beware duds!

## Things We Do That Aren't So Smart for Sleep

The habits of modern life are often not conducive to getting good sleep. Beyond all the work, home, and social scheduling pressures, there are screens, food, and exercise that get in the way. Exercising too late can disrupt sleep and eating heavy meals too late can do the same. And then, there are screens. From the overview of chronobiology, you will recognise that **light** matters. It delays the onset of melatonin release from the brain, and even dim light (~10lux) will do that. A modestly lit room is around

xii. A downloadable sleep log can be found at the Sleep Foundation, https://www.sleepfoundation.org/sample-sleep-log.

200lux, and a bedside lamp is somewhere between 20 and 80lux. Then there's blue light – the type that comes from our phones, computers, and tablets. Reading on a tablet suppresses melatonin release by 50%, and the resulting shift of timing of melatonin release causes negative effects the next day, essentially like jet lag – that hungover feeling.

When we sleep, our core body temperature drops, and indeed in order to *get* to sleep our temperature needs to drop by ~1° C. This is helped by the **ambient temperature** of the room not being too high, and yet many will seek to have warm bedrooms. The ideal temperature is said to be 18–18.5° C.

The effects of **diet** on sleep can vary between individuals, but there are a few things that apply to us all. As mentioned, a heavy meal soon before bed disturbs sleep. Severe calorie restriction (e.g., 800 kcal/day or less) also has negative impacts on sleep. Eating a high carbohydrate, low fat diet for a few days leads to reduced non-REM (deep) sleep, increased REM (dreamy) sleep, and more awakenings, compared to a low carbohydrate and high fat diet.[257]

Although many assume that **alcohol** aids sleep, its effects are not beneficial in this respect.[258] Higher doses have more significant negative effects: although it makes a person fall asleep quicker, the sleep is disrupted with more awakenings and shorter total duration of sleep, less REM, and more non-REM sleep. Even drinking alcohol six hours before bed-time (i.e., happy hour) disrupts sleep even though there is no alcohol left in the brain by that time.[259] At lower doses there can be initial stimulating effects in the first hour, such that sleep latency is delayed in that time frame. With increasing amounts of alcohol (e.g., moderate intake of two to three units),[xiii] the sedating effects become more apparent. However, a few hours later as the blood alcohol level falls, there is a rebound, with frequent awakenings and a rise in stress hormones called catecholamines.

xiii. These units refer to the UK standard of 10 ml (8 grams) of pure alcohol per unit (https://en.wikipedia.org/wiki/Standard_drink).

| | | |
|---|---|---|
| **Social life** | **Nutrition** | **Schedule** (early starts/late finishes) |
| **Culture** | **Health** | **Worries** |
| **Family** | **Exercise** | **Screen-time** |
| **Environment** | **Mood** | **Hydration** |
| **Caffeine** | **Chronotype** | **Alcohol** |

**Table 17.5** Factors that commonly affect sleep.

## The Effects of Insufficient Sleep on Performance

The effects on the brain of insufficient sleep, or 'sleep deprivation' (which just means less than seven hours/night) are many and profound. Insufficient sleep results in declines in brain activation, especially in those areas sustaining executive control: higher cognition, alertness, situational awareness, and memory capacity.[260] Short-term memory is significantly impaired even after one night of reduced sleep, and those who have not slept for one night are eight times more likely to have attention lapses than those who have slept for eight hours. Furthermore, even those who achieve six hours sleep per night demonstrate significantly greater cognitive impairment compared to those who achieve eight hours or more.[261]

The impact of these findings can be catastrophic if we consider the effects on those who have to make critical decisions and act on them when they have had limited sleep – e.g., doctors, air traffic controllers, military personnel. In the field of clinical medicine, sleep deprivation results in a reported 20% increase in surgical errors and 14% more time needed to perform procedures, significant impairment in interpreting routine investigations, and poorer outcomes in performance in higher qualification examinations.[262]

In 1997 Dawson and Reid published a study of forty subjects who participated in two counterbalanced experiments.[263] In one they were kept awake for twenty-eight hours (from 8:00 a.m. until 12:00 noon the following day), and in the other they consumed 10–15 g alcohol at thirty-minute intervals from 8:00 a.m. until their mean blood alcohol concentration reached 0.10%. Brain and motor function ('cognitive psychomotor performance') were measured at half-hour intervals using a computer-administered test of hand-eye coordination (an unpredictable tracking task). The results showed that being awake for at least eighteen hours has the same effects as having a blood content (BAC) of 0.05%. Being awake for at least twenty-four hours is equal to having a blood alcohol content of 0.10%. A BAC of above 0 is illegal in many countries, a limit of 0.02 is common. In the USA and England 0.08% is illegal. Clearly, sleep deprivation makes us unsafe.

## Sleep, Learning, and Memory

Earlier in this book, elements of learning, apprenticeship, and development of mastery and expertise were described (chapter 3). Sleep has a significant impact on these; it can make or break the learning process. Many studies have demonstrated that sleep after learning enhances retention. Take for example a study of two groups, both trained in a finger tapping motor skill, one trained at 10:00 p.m. and retested the next morning after twelve hours of sleep, and then tested again twelve hours later (Sleep First).[264] The second group was trained in the morning and retested that evening after twelve hours of being awake, and again the next day (Wake First). Performances were significantly better after sleep: for those who trained at night then slept (Sleep First), their motor performance improved by a significant 21%. When tested later in that day after twelve hours of being awake, they had not improved much more. In those who were trained in the morning and tested that evening after twelve hours of being awake (Wake First), they showed no significant improvement, but again after a nights' sleep they showed a 19% improvement on testing the next morning. Further analysis revealed that when the night of sleep was divided into quarters, overnight motor skill improvement was correlated to the proportion of stage 2 non-REM sleep in the fourth quarter of the sleep period. Hence sleep, and in particular non-REM sleep, plays a role in learning and motor skills: *we need sleep to learn,* and poor sleep will seriously impair learning and the effectiveness of deliberate practice.

## Effects of Insufficient Sleep on Athletic Performance

Although those who physically train heavily tend to need more sleep to recover, the sleep habits and sleep patterns of athletes are often poor. Research indicates that 50–78% of elite athletes experience sleep disturbance and 22–26% suffer highly disturbed sleep. Elite athletes have been shown to have shorter sleep duration and poorer sleep quality compared with their non-athletic peers. This can relate to the negative impacts of heavy training (especially overtraining) on sleep, along with the many other general causes of sleep disturbance that apply to us all.

Sleep deprivation results in impaired reaction times, and in sport this is often the difference between success and failure, and injury or health. Consider the significant implications of sleep deprivation for injury susceptibility. One study of young athletes has shown a rise in incidence of injury from ~17% in those getting nine hours of sleep per night, to 70–75% in those getting just six hours.[265] Athletes who slept on average less than eight hours per night were 1.7 times more likely to have had an injury compared with athletes who slept for eight or more hours.

| Hours of sleep/night | Cumulative incidence of injuries over a 21-month period |
|---|---|
| 6 | 70–75% |
| 7 | 60% |
| 8 | 35% |
| 9 | 17–18% |

**Table 17.6** Estimates of the risk of sustaining injuries in sport increases significantly in those who are sleep deprived.[266]

Less sleep impairs the ability to sustain exercise and also results in poorer performance in training, and indeed, teams who sleep better are more successful in competition.[267] The only element of performance where there is no evidence of sleep deprivation having an impact is peak muscle strength, but in most circumstances the overwhelming effects on all other aspects of performance means this is of little comfort.

## The Benefits of Napping

*'Think what a better world it would be if we all, the whole world, had cookies and milk about three o'clock every afternoon and then lay down on our blankets for a nap'.*

**Barbara Jordan**[xiv]

Famous nappers include JFK, Einstein, Napoleon, and Churchill, and whether they knew it or not, planned napping is a smart way of enhancing performance. Napping not only helps to make up for any sleep 'debt' left from the night before; even those who sleep well will benefit.[268] A short nap can raise our alertness, cognitive skills, and motor performance. A study at NASA on sleep in military pilots and astronauts found that a forty-minute nap improved performance by 34% and alertness by 100%.[269] Several premier soccer teams and other elite sports teams have napping facilities for their athletes as part of their performance plan, which isn't surprising when research has shown that twenty- to thirty-minute naps not only improve reaction times and alertness, but also other physical performance markers like sprint and peak jump velocity performance.[270] Naps should be timed for the part of the day when we are beginning to slump, and for most people that is in the afternoon; the nap should not be left until too late in the day because it may interfere with night-time sleep. The time includes around five to seven minutes to get to

xiv. American civil rights lawyer.

sleep, plus the fifteen- to twenty-minute nap. Many find it difficult to nap initially; it takes a little planning (when, where), and it also takes practice. In night-shift work, just as in the day, breaks for twenty- to thirty-minute naps have been shown to improve performance.[271]

## Sleep Desynchronization: Jet Lag and Shift Work

Travelling punishes the body and the brain, and jet lag and night shifts put us on the wrong side of our body clocks. When we travel across two or more time zones, the time shift means that our circadian rhythms are out of sync with the time of day in our new time zone; our master clock is telling us to sleep, eat, and function at the wrong 'new' time of day. Our internal clocks will adjust over the course of a few days: one day for every hour difference. Typically, it is harder to adjust when we travel east. Night-shift work is like an extreme form of jet lag, flipping our natural circadian rhythms, and is even worse if the individual cycles between different shift times, especially between night and day shifts.

When travelling, even the process of being confined in a small space to travel, and sleep deprivation after travelling, leaves our bodies slower and more prone to injury. In sport, jet lag appears to have a significant effect on performance in most situations. The effects of sleep loss and the impact of travel on muscle elasticity, speed, power, reaction times, alertness, cognition, and balance can be significant, even without the individual being aware they are 'out of sync'. Just look at how time zone changes may even affect winning percentages. For example, in the NCAA Basketball League, the winning percentage for teams traveling from the west to the east drops by 38% when they are crossing two or more time zones.[272] Aiming to arrive some days before competition is prudent, although even in high performance sport this is frequently not adhered to.

Earlier I described how our internal clocks respond to light as a principal regulator of our body rhythms and wakefulness. The use of light to mitigate the effects of jet lag can be very effective. Since our internal clocks are largely regulated by light, seeking light to help us adjust to new daytime hours and the use of artificial lighting are both useful approaches. For the latter, lighting that is shifted towards the blue end of the spectrum (closest to daylight) is particularly helpful and can be used as a strategy for night-shift workers. Blue light, though, has negative effects as well, as discussed earlier.

Fortunately, light is not the only factor that influences sleep; food, exercise, and temperature also can help (and are the principal mechanisms for people who are blind). We can use all of these triggers to facilitate early adjustment to our new time zone. Seasoned, successful travellers who perform well at their destination are those who learn how to manage the physiological challenges involved.

Consider also the role of exercise as a tool for jet lag. Exercising *either* at 7 a.m. *or* between 1 p.m. and 4 p.m. shifts the circadian rhythm to an earlier time (helpful for those who travel east). Engaging in exercise between 7 p.m. and 10 p.m. pushes the body clock back (helpful if going west).[273] Age or sex does not affect these results, and seemingly exercising at other times does not significantly affect body clocks. Note that the first workout we do on the day of arrival should be light to moderate in intensity and volume and should be preceded by warmup and flexibility work, since soft tissues are stiff and more injury prone after travel.

There are, of course, other things that can help us to deal with the effects of jet lag. Many of us will automatically reach for caffeine to help, because it is a central nervous stimulant. Coffee or tea are the best sources as they also contain a range of antioxidants that are beneficial to health; a cup of filter coffee has 95–200 mg caffeine. Doses of 225–600 mg have been recommended in relation to jet lag. However in some (especially those who are lightweight and/or not habitual coffee drinkers), even a 75 mg serving of caffeine can increase attention and alertness, and doses of 160–600 mg can improve alertness and speed reasoning and memory. The effects typically wear off within three to four hours.

For shift workers, it is better to consume regular, small doses of caffeine and taper off halfway through the shift. For any of us, if taken within four to six hours of bedtime, sleep quality will be impaired, sleep latency can be prolonged, and overall sleep duration reduced. Research has also shown that caffeine and L-theanine (an amino acid found in black and green tea) synergistically promote alertness, attention, and task completion, especially in the first hour after ingestion.

Beyond exercise, sleep timing consistency, and limiting caffeine and blue light in the evening, there are a few other strategies to assist with sleep. The first is food, starting with tryptophan, which is found in milk, meat, fish, poultry, eggs, beans, peanuts, cheese, and leafy green vegetables. A decrease in tryptophan levels in the blood has been shown to produce sleep disturbances.[274] Tryptophan is converted to serotonin in the brain and serotonin is converted into melatonin, which as you will recall influences the sleep-wake cycle. Having a sleep friendly snack, typically rich in tryptophan, can aid sleep. Although high protein snacks cause restlessness at night, high glycaemic index carbohydrate snacks (though not encouraged in general), can aid sleep onset through making tryptophan more available to the brain. One study has shown that a high GI meal provided four hours before bedtime shortened sleep onset latency by 48.6% compared with a low GI meal. The high GI meal was much more effective when consumed four hours before bedtime compared with consumption one hour before bedtime.[275]

Heavy meals late at night may not be avoidable but have negative sleep impacts. For example, consider observed sleep patterns during Ramadan, when eating only occurs after sunset every day for twenty-nine to thirty days. A significant delay in sleep onset is noted, along with an increase in body temperature at night, increased cortisol (stress hormone) concentrations, and reduced slow wave sleep and REM sleep. Energy restriction (e.g., on low calorie diets) can also have similar negative impacts on sleep.

A very popular sleep aid is melatonin. In spite of the fact that this is a powerful hormone, and in some countries is classified as a drug, it is available over the counter as a supplement in some countries, including the USA. It may be useful in some clinical sleep disorders, which is beyond the scope of this book. Melatonin has a use in managing jet lag, but in fact the evidence for its effectiveness in this respect is limited, and there is likely a placebo effect. Generally, if melatonin is used, it should be taken after arrival at the destination, although if travelling eastward it may help to take it on the day of travel at the ideal bedtime in the destination time zone, particularly if crossing five or more time zones.

Another common sleep supplement in use is valerian. This is a herb that is considered to have a calming effect on the nervous system, and a subjective improvement in sleep quality with its use is reported.[276] Side effects can include drowsiness the next day, dizziness, and allergic reaction. Furthermore, it may influence growth hormone release, which may have health implications and also contraindicates its use by athletes as it represents a doping violation.

Perhaps at this late stage of this book, it is suitable to close the chapter with words from Homer's Odyssey: '*There is a time for many words, and there is also a time for sleep*'.

## Key Messages:

- Sleep is not a luxury. It is key to a healthier, happier, and longer life, and to achieving goals.
- A lack of consistent, good-quality sleep significantly impairs performance, and so it is imperative to consider sleep as a priority in the journey to achieving goals.
- Being rigorous about good sleep behaviours and protecting against the many elements in life that can threaten sleep seem obvious steps to take to enhance our well-being and performance, and yet this approach is all too often overlooked.
- Sleep monitoring technologies can be extremely valuable in improving insights into an individual's night-time health. Subjective evaluation of sleep quality, and logging of activities that may influence sleep (e.g., eating and screen behaviours) also offers valuable information.

# 18

# Technologies in Human Performance

## Useful Servants but Dangerous Masters

Technologies have changed the world and continue to do so, for better or for worse, in almost every domain of life. The tech craze has been overwhelming, with new tools appearing every day, some of which have become widely – and rapidly – accepted in day-to-day life. Bill Gates is quoted as saying, 'The advance of technology is based on making it fit in so that you don't really even notice it, so it's part of daily life'. How true this has proven to be – but some of the acceptance of technologies has been without foundation. Only now is the world starting to realise the implications of this 'boom', the need to scrutinise the products we are using and their roles, usefulness, and dangers on a personal and societal level.

As in other areas of life, technologies play a central role in human performance programmes on both individual and organisational levels.

While it may already feel like a tech-saturated world, in truth the field is in its infancy, though it is growing at an exponential rate. We have digital health technologies that offer opportunities to diagnose, understand, and treat diseases earlier and more effectively, body-worn and home devices that assist the individual with monitoring their vitality and ability to perform even day-to-day tasks more easily, tools that allow the development of specific skills across many domains, performance analysis systems in sport and the workplace where the individual's every movement and heartbeat can be tracked and analysed, and machine learning and 'artificial intelligence' systems that can provide insights into how and why we human beings behave and respond as we do.

| Type of tool | Examples of outputs |
| --- | --- |
| **Body-worn devices, chips, clothing, home systems** | Various vitality-related markers including: heart rate and rhythm derived metrics, fitness markers, sweat, body temperature, oxygen levels, movement metrics, biomechanics, body composition, balance, alertness, reaction times, work load, sleep, energy expenditure, glucose levels, *stress, *recovery, *strain, *readiness. |
| **Computer vision technologies (e.g., via static cameras, drones)** | Movement, biomechanics, technique, training/competition performance and strategy analysis, equipment design. |
| **Sonar, GPS** | Movement, biomechanics, training/competition performance and strategy analysis |
| **Virtual reality environments** | Skills acquisition and situational training. |
| **Machine learning** | Prediction of performance, injuries, illnesses |
| **Equipment advances, monitoring systems within equipment and clothes** | Injury prevention, performance improvement |

**Table 18.1** Examples of technologies in human performance.

* Blanket terms used by tech companies in their products.

The concerns relating to the regulation of technologies in human performance have been highlighted in chapter 2, and the importance of this issue cannot be over-emphasised. Some users at governmental, organisational, and individual levels have yet to become 'savvy' as to how they select tools to use, and this should be the next stage in the evolution of how we choose to use technologies to ensure they improve our lives. Technologies should not be optimised for those who develop them; they must be optimised for those who are responsible for how they are used, and for the users themselves. Those professionals who choose to use and recommend new tools must act with scientific rigour and responsibility to ensure the tools are valid. With that comes the need for these professionals – whether they be clinicians using digital health tools, coaches in sport, or advisers and leaders in the corporate sector – to understand the tools they are using, the data that are derived from them, potential pitfalls in measurement and interpretation, and the best methods of providing feedback and actions from the information gained. This in itself represents an enormous challenge.[277]

When one considers the challenges that even highly qualified 'experts' have with fully understanding the technologies available in the human performance field, it is no surprise that the individual user who, for example, is choosing a device to monitor their health and assist them with enhancing their vitality, can find it extremely challenging to know that the tool they are choosing is valid. The best tools will be underpinned by honesty and transparency by those who produce them. Much is yet to be achieved by the tech sector in this respect. While concerns are so often raised about our reliance on technologies, this would be far less of an issue if we learn to judge their quality and place more effectively. For that to be realistic, those who produce these technologies must provide the user with the information in clear and simple forms. It is clear that resources are needed for users to access advice, support, and evidence-based recommendations for the best technologies to support their health and performance to ensure they make the best choices. Taking an example from healthcare, sites have been developed to support digital health tools, providing resources for patients on recommended digital interventions, support to troubleshoot devices, and access to testing health apps and

| | |
|---|---|
| **Validity** | Do the outputs reflect relevant markers? |
| **Relevance** | Is the tool relevant and useful to the specific user? |
| **Reliability and Accuracy** | What is the tool's reliability and accuracy across different populations and under different circumstances? |
| **Scientific Evidence** | Are there independently published reports to support its use? |
| **Added Value** | Is there added value to using the tool? |
| **Feedback** | Does the tool provide feedback that can be easily interpreted? |
| **Resources** | What are the available resources that offer updates, support, and troubleshooting for the tool? |

**Table 18.2** Some essential criteria to selecting a performance tool.

devices. Other systems are being developed elsewhere.[278] Such a template could be applied to performance technologies as a whole.

Lastly, advances in equipment due to technologies must also be highlighted. This is a huge subject in itself and outside of the focus in this book. Nevertheless, of all the advances that technologies have brought to high performance sport, this aspect is perhaps the most obvious. Developments in golf clubs are largely the reason why professionals now routinely hit the ball forty yards farther than they did twenty years ago, and indeed such modifications have changed (and some would say threaten) the game. Similar improvements in tennis, squash, and badminton racquets are also clear examples. Such advances have also contributed to greater safety: headgear in rugby and American football to reduce concussion, cushioning and stability technologies in footwear to reduce injuries, bicycle saddle technologies to protect soft tissues, customised protective eyewear and jaw guards to protect facial structures, alterations in racing car systems to protect drivers... the list is lengthy. Many such technologies have inbuilt sensors to monitor effectiveness and identify trauma. These technologies are contributing to enhancing the safety of many sports in an era where many of these activities are being recognised as having inherent dangers to the individuals involved.

There is no doubt that furthering our understanding of human performance across all domains in life will be fuelled by innovative technologies that provide insight into the effects of training, environments, and day-to-day stresses on human beings and their function. When there are so many opportunities, there is a huge hunger for tools that make challenging performance journeys easier, and perhaps as a result an over-optimistic tendency to use products without judging them properly first. Amongst all the excitement and in spite of the pressures to deliver results, we must all learn to channel technologies carefully and be rigorous in how we select the right tool for the specific needs of the individual user. In that way technologies will serve us well.

*The future is still so much bigger than the past.*

**Tim Berners-Lee, inventor of the world wide web**

# 19

# Looking to the Horizon

It is testament to your powers of perseverance that you have reached the final stages of this book, and hopefully you are enlightened by the insights provided and perhaps even more curious about the keys to human performance than when you started. The challenges in writing about such an immense topic are obvious, because the subject encompasses the entirety of how we function as individuals; how we react and respond to the challenges we face, to our environments, and to different situations; and how we interact with others. The focus of this book has been on the individual rather than teams, for sensible reasons. The factors that influence team performance start with the individuals within it, and the additional aspects that apply to teams are perhaps a subject for another book.

Any text that seeks to embrace such a huge field, to provide a holistic view of the essentials of human performance, will inevitably have some loose ends. A lengthy book could be written about every single subject in each chapter, but that was not the goal. I hope the contents of the book have not only provided insights, but have also inspired curiosity and triggered more questions and a desire to learn more. In your further reading, just remember the criteria for safely assessing information and tools that have been recommended.

The field of human performance is informed by research in areas that include physiology, neuroscience, medicine, behavioural sciences, psychology, biomechanics, and technologies, and our insights are changing with every week that passes. There will therefore always be loose ends, and new directions that deserve attention. To serve this purpose, updates with information about progress, research, and innovation in the field will continue to be provided on my website: ***www.highperformer.co.uk***.

The journey to further understanding how we perform, and what makes us thrive, will always continue.

# Appendix

## BMI

The American Cancer Society's BMI calculator is available at: https://www.cancer.org/healthy/eat-healthy-get-active/take-control-your-weight/body-mass-index-bmi-calculator.html. The site stresses that 'if you are overweight or obese, even a small weight loss (10% of your current weight) can lower your risk of several diseases. People who are overweight or obese have a greater chance of developing several types of cancer – including colorectal cancer and breast cancer (for women past menopause) – as well as high blood pressure, high blood cholesterol or other lipid disorders, diabetes, heart disease, and stroke'.

## Waist Circumference

Waist circumference is a good measurement to assess whether you are likely to have a lot of visceral fat. It is measured by wrapping a tape measure around the waist midpoint between the bottom of your ribs and top of your hips, typically just above the belly button. The British Heart Foundation offers a calculator where you can determine your risk level: https://extras.bhf.org.uk/patientinfo/waist-measurement_v1.0/app.

From a practical perspective, because they are easy to measure, you can monitor progress with a programme by combining BMI with waist circumference using these tools. If possible, get your skinfolds measured routinely by a trained individual or consider using smart scales, which allow you to measure your body fat in the comfort of your own home.

# Glossary

**andragogy** – learning by adults

**amygdala** – the part of the brain that influences emotions

**basal metabolic rate** (BMR) – the rate of our metabolism at rest

**body mass index** (BMI) – a person's weight divided by their height squared ($kg/m^2$)

**burnout** – extreme exhaustion, lack of well-being, inability to cope, reduced performance, and major health issues

**cardiometabolic** – a combination of heart and metabolism, typically relating to diseases that affect both, such as diabetes

**cardiovascular** – heart and blood vessels

**chronobiology** – literally 'time biology', the timing of our biological rhythms

**chrono-nutrition** – coordinating food intake with the circadian body rhythm (i.e., the internal biological clock)

**chronotype** – a person's natural inclination with regard to the times of day when they prefer to sleep or when they are most alert, energetic, or creative

**circadian rhythm** – a biological internal process that regulates the sleep-wake cycle and repeats approximately every twenty-four hours

**cognition** – mental processes that include thinking, knowing, remembering, judging, perception, planning, and problem solving

**conscientiousness** – being goal orientated, disciplined, organised, and diligent

**cortex** – the thinking part of the brain

**endocannabinoids** – chemicals produced by the body that are also found in cannabis

**dopamine** – the pleasure-seeking chemical that drives the brain's reward pathway

**eustress** – positive stress

**executive function** – a set of mental skills that include working memory (a form of short-term memory we use to perform tasks), flexible thinking, and self-control

**expertise** – mastery that translates to concrete, consistent, repeatable performances that are above and beyond what our peers achieve

**flow state** – being fully immersed in the process, fully focused and in control, energised, and enjoying the activity

**frontal lobe** – the part of the brain where executive functions, thinking, emotions, impulse and behavioural control, personality, and motor skills are controlled; includes the pre-frontal cortex

**fronto-parietal** – a combination of the formal and parietal lobes of the brain

**functional Magnetic Resonance Imaging** (fMRI) – a form of imaging of the brain that shows areas of brain activity by detecting changes associated with blood flow

**ghrelin** – the 'hunger hormone' that stimulates appetite but also has other effects on health

**glycaemic index** (GI) – an indicator of how quickly an insulin spike will occur after we eat, and how much of a sugar 'high' and 'low' follows

**glycaemic load** (GL) – glycaemic index x grams of carbohydrate in the meal

**habit** – a routine or practice performed regularly; an automatic response to a specific situation

**health** – a state of complete physical, mental, and social well-being, and not merely the absence of disease or infirmity

**holistic** – whole, or whole person

**homeostasis** – the process of maintaining a stable internal environment in the body, for optimal functioning

**hypothalamus** – a region of the brain that coordinates body processes including body temperature, thirst, hunger, and other systems, and is also involved in sleep and emotional activity

**learning curve** – the rate of a person's progress in gaining experience or new skills

**leptin** – a hormone released from the fat cells that sends signals to the brain and helps to control satiety after eating

**lipids** – fats and oils, including cholesterol

**mastery** – having a comprehensive knowledge or skill in a particular subject or activity

**metacognition** – literally 'beyond' or 'higher order' thinking; conscious self-monitoring

**microbiome** – the genetic material of all the microbes – bacteria, fungi, protozoa, and viruses – that live on and inside the human body

**mindfulness** – conscious awareness of the moment and our responses to it; knowing what is going on inside and outside ourselves, moment by moment

**motivation** – the internal and/or external forces that produce the initiation, direction, intensity, and persistence of behaviour

**neurones** – nerve cells

**neuroplasticity** – the ability of the brain to form and reorganize synaptic connections

**neuromotor** (or **neuromuscular**) – the effects of nerve impulses on muscles

**parietal lobe** – the part of the brain where perception, information processing, and body position are controlled

**passion** – a strong inclination towards a self-defining activity (or object) that one likes (or even loves), finds important and meaningful, and in which one invests time and energy

**perfectionism** – a trait of having unrealistically high expectations and overly critical self-evaluations

**perseverance** – persistence, continued effort, and determination even in the face of setbacks

**performance mindset** – reflecting a positive way of thinking about things; a set of attitudes that influence our decision making and approach; a set of beliefs that reflect how we see ourselves, our intelligence, our talents, and our capabilities

**prefrontal cortex** – the part of the brain in the frontal lobe that is the headquarters for executive control

**pressure** – our responses to an expectation, often self-imposed, to perform well in a situation

**recovery** – restoring the body and mind to a replenished state

**self-awareness** – seeing ourselves clearly; how we think, react, and behave

**self-efficacy** – our belief in our ability to perform well in specific areas of life and to apply the necessary behaviours to achieve specific goals

**sleep** – a reversible behavioural state of perceptual disengagement from, and unresponsiveness to, the environment

**stress** – the body's physiological, emotional, and mental reactions to feeling threatened, triggered by one or more stressors in our environment

**synapses** – connections between nerves

ultradian rhythms – recurrent cycles that are shorter than circadian rhythms

**vitality** – aliveness; the product of our physical, physiological, mental, and emotional states; whole-person performance fitness

**working memory** – a form of short-term memory we use to perform tasks

## List of Figures

**3** The Apprenticeship Journey.

**3.1** The journey to mastery and expertise.

**3.2** Ingredients of mastery: Knowledge, motor skills, reasoning/judgement, experience.

**3.3** The four lobes of the brain and their principal functions. (Executive function is based in the prefrontal cortex of the brain.)

**3.4** The principal components of executive function, representing essential skills to perform in every domain of life.

**3.5** Number of years to reach 10,000 hours of deliberate practice, based on practicing 5 days per week, 46 weeks/year.

**3.6** The most successful chess players have put in significantly more hours of practice.

**3.7** Six Key Characteristics of Performance drive the development of mastery and expertise.

**3.8** Learning curves vary significantly across individuals and tasks.

**3.9** How the learning process may feel to the learner if planning is inadequate and/or expectations are not managed.

### 6 Passion for the Purpose

**6.1** Features of passion.

### 7 Perseverance

**7.1** Components of motivation.

**7.2** Motivation and the hierarchy of needs.

**7.3** Factors that influence intrinsic motivation.

### 8 Conscientiousness

**8.1** Features of conscientiousness.

**8.2** Components of executive function.

**8.3** Health benefits of conscientiousness.

**8.4** Dopamine pathways in the brain.

**8.5** The habit loop.

**8.6** Steps towards creating a new habit.

## 9 Self-Efficacy

**9.1** Factors that influence self-efficacy.

## 10 Self-Awareness

**10.1** Self-awareness: Conscious self-monitoring.

**10.2** The Johari Window and modelling approaches to enhancing self-awareness.

## 11 Vitality

**11.1** Components of Vitality.

**11.2** The acute stress response.

**11.3** The principal physiological changes in the body when exposed to acute stress.

**11.4** The human function curve: Some stress has positive effects on performance, but getting the right balance is key.

## 12 Chronogiology

**12.1** The master clock.

**12.2** The best times of the day for Larks and Third Birds to perform specific things, based on chronobiology. (Owls typically peak in cognitive tasks in the latter part of the day and are more create late morning.)

**12.3** The focus/recovery task performance cycle.

## 13 Fitness

**13.1** Balancing training load to optimise gains. (Optimal load varies across individuals and changes with time and fitness.)

**13.2** Lack of recovery after imposed loads can result in overtraining, underperformance, illnesses, and injuries.

**13.3** Some of the benefits of regular aerobic exercise on the body.

**13.4** Benefits of exercise on metabolism and performance.

**13.5** Some of the effects of acute exercise on the brain.

**13.6** Exercise benefits the brain through a number of mechanisms.

**13.7** Duration of effects after at least 30 minutes moderate to vigorous cardiovascular exercise on the brain. More vigorous exercise seems to have greater effects.

**13.8** Our circadian rhythm influences our physical performance.

## 14 Fitness in the High Performance Athlete

**14.1** Typical aerobic capacities (VO2max) of elite athletes in different sports.

## 15 Nutrition for Us All

**15.1** Important considerations relating to nutrition for performance.

**15.2** An example of the way individuals burn energy through their BMR, dietary thermogenesis, and physical activity.

**15.3** How blood glucose spikes and falls with food of low and high GI values.

**15.4** The brain-gut axis has a major influence on how we perform.

**15.5** Contribution of carbohydrate and fat to energy at different exercise intensities.

**15.6** Circadian clocks and their effects.

## 17 Sleep to Succeed

**17.1** Sleep homeostat.

**17.2** Melatonin, cortisol, and core body temperature changes across the 24-hour sleep-wake cycle.

**17.3** The sleep hypnogram: Each sleep cycle lasts about 90 minutes and consists of different sleep stages.

# List of Tables


## 4 What Kind of Learner Are You?

**4.1** VARK learning styles.

## 6 Passion for the Purpose

**6.1** Correlation between passion and other factors.

## 8 Conscientiousness

**8.1** Features of high and low levels of conscientiousness.

## 9 Self-Efficacy

**9.1** Steps towards optimising self-efficacy.

## 10 Self-Awareness

**10.1** Examples of the benefits of self-awareness.

**10.2** Self-awareness is a result of our understanding of insights into our own selves (internal self-awareness) and how much we understand how others see us (external self-awareness).

## 11 Vitality

**11.1** Characteristics of those with a high performance mindset.

**11.2** Necessary requirements to achieve a flow state.

## 13 Fitness

**13.1** The five components of physical fitness.

**13.2** Classification of exercise intensity based on heart rate reserve (HRR) and rated perceived exertion (RPE).

**13.3** How to calculate Heart Rate Reserve.

**13.4** Evidence-based benefits of CV and resistance exercise.

**13.5** An example of exercise session types for a reasonably fit person across a week of fitness training.

**13.6** Basic physical health measurements that relate to both health and performance.

**13.7** Basic blood tests that relate to health and performance (to be interpreted by a physician).

**13.8** Examples of performance-related fitness tests.

**13.9** Cardiovascular fitness: Maximum oxygen uptake (VO2max) standards in the male general population.

**13.10** VO2 max standards in the female general population.

## 14 Fitness in the High Performance Athlete

**14.1** Vertical jump height reference standards.

## 15 Nutrition for Us All

**15.1** Body Mass Index (BMI) categories.

**15.2** Percentage body fat in different groups.

**15.3** Calculation of BMR using the Henry Equation.

**15.4** How to calculate total daily calorie needs.

**15.5** Glycaemic index and load ranges.

**15.6** Associations between components of vitality and the gut microbiome.

**15.7** Examples of the effects of high sugar intake.

**15.8** The Mediterranean diet.

**15.9** Percentages of calories derived from carbohydrate, protein, and fat in different diets.

## 16 Nutrition for Exercise and Recovery

**16.1** Examples of healthy recovery snacks.

**16.2** Carbohydrate intake for specific training purposes.

**16.3** Tips to achieving lower body fat.

## 17 Sleep to Succeed

**17.1** Some consequences of insufficient sleep.

**17.2** Loss of productivity due to sleep loss across 5 OECD countries.

**17.3** Important dimensions of sleep.

**17.4** A description of sleep stages.

**17.5** Factors that commonly affect sleep.

**17.6** Estimates of the risk of sustaining injuries in sport increases significantly in those who are sleep deprived.

## 18 Technologies in Human Performance

**18.1** Examples of technologies in human performance.

**18.2** Some essential criteria to selecting a performance tool.

# Endnotes

## 1. Predicting Performance


1. The Free Dictionary, s.v. 'performing', https://www.thefreedictionary.com/performing.

2. Beth McGroarty, 'Wellness Industry Statistics & Facts', Global Wellness Institute, October 2018, https://globalwellnessinstitute.org/press-room/statistics-and-facts.

3. BusinessWire, 'Global Corporate Wellness Market to Surpass US$100.0 Billion by 2027—Coherent Market Insights', 4 September 2019, https://www.businesswire.com/news/home/20190904005539/en/Global-Corporate-Wellness-Market-to-Surpass-US-100.0-Billion-by-2027-%E2%80%93-Coherent-Market-Insights.

4. CISION PR Newswire, 'Digital Health Market Size to Reach USD 385.8 Billion by 2025: Valutes Reports', 23 April 2020, https://www.prnewswire.co.uk/news-releases/digital-health-market-size-to-reach-usd-385-8-billion-by-2025-valuates-reports-826205814.html.

5. CISION PR Newswire, 'Digital Health Market Size'.

6. A Bandura, 'Self-efficacy: Toward a unifying theory of behavioral change', *Psychological Review* 84, no. 2 (1977): 191–215; A Bandura, *Social Foundations of Thought and Action: A Social Cognitive Theory* (Englewood Cliffs, NJ: Prentice-Hall, 1986); A Bandura, 'Social cognitive theory of self-regulation', *Organizational Behavior and Human Decision Processes* 50 (1991): 248–57; A Bandura, *Self-Efficacy: The Exercise of Control* (New York: Freeman, 1997).


## 2. Notes of Caution


7. Wikipedia, s.v. 'Black box', last edited 26 December 2020, https://en.wikipedia.org/wiki/Black_box.

8. Stefan Pertz, *The Guru in Me: Critical Perspectives on Management* (Munich: GRIN Verlag, 2013), 2–3.

9. Joel Mlecko, 'The Guru in Hindu Tradition', *Numen* 29, no. 1 (1982): 33–61.

10. A L Sellier, I Scopelliti, and C K Morewedge, 'Debiasing training improves decision making in the field', *Psychological Science* 30, no. 9 (2019): 1371–79.


## 3. The Apprenticeship Journey


11. K A Ericsson, 'Why expert performance is special and cannot be extrapolated from studies of performance in the general population: A response to criticisms', *Intelligence* 45 (2014): 81–103.

12. K Johnston et al., 'Talent Identification in sport: a systematic review', *Sports Medicine* 48 (2018): 97–109.

13. K A Ericsson and K W Harwell, 'Deliberate practice and proposed limits on the effects of practice on the acquisition of expert performance: Why the original definition matters and recommendations for future research', *Frontiers in Psychology* 10 (2019): 2396.

14. J R Andrews-Hanna et al. 'Disruption of large-scale brain systems in advanced aging', *Neuron* 56, no. 5 (6 December 2007): 924–35.

15. R Cabeza, N D Anderson, J K Locantore, and A R McIntosh, 'Aging gracefully: compensatory brain activity in high-performing older adults', *Neuroimage* 17, no. 3 (November 2002): 1394–402; D C Park, P Reuter-Lorenz, 'The adaptive brain: Aging and neurocognitive scaffolding', *Annual Review of Psychology* 60 (2009): 173–96, doi:10.1146/annurev.psych.59.103006.093656.

16. J Zuk, C Benjamin, A Kenyon, and N Gaab, 'Behavioral and neural correlates of executive functioning in musicians and non-musicians', *PLoS One* 9, no. 6 (2014): e99868.

17. T Lesiuk, J A Bugos, and B Murakami, 'A rationale for music training to enhance executive functions in Parkinson's disease: An overview of the problem', *Healthcare* 6, no. 2 (2018): 35, doi:10.3390/healthcare6020035.

18. E A Maguire et al., 'Navigation-related structural change in the hippocampi of taxi drivers', *PNAS* 97, no. 8 (11 April 2000): 4398–403.

19. E A Maguire, E R Valentine, J M Wilding, and N Kapur, 'Routes to remembering: The brains behind superior memory', *Nature Neuroscience* 6 (2003): 90–95; K Woollett, H J Spiers, and E J Maguire, 'Talent in the taxi: A model system for exploring expertise' *Philosophical Transactions* 364 (2009): 1407–16.

20. L Zamarian, A Ischebeck, and M Delazer, 'Neuroscience of learning arithmetic—evidence from brain imaging studies', *Neuroscience and Biobehavioral Reviews* 33 (2009): 909–25.

21. K Yarrow, P Brown, and J Krakauer, 'Inside the brain of an elite athlete: The neural processes that support high achievement in sports', *Nature Reviews Neuroscience* 10 (2009): 585–96.

22. R N Haber and L Haber, 'Perception and attention during low-altitude high-speed flight', in *Principles and Practice of Aviation Psychology*, ed. P S Tsang and M A Vidulich (Mahwah, NJ: Erlbaum, 2003), 21–68.

23. R E Roberts et al., 'Expert cognitive control and individual differences associated with frontal and parietal white matter microstructure', *Journal of Neuroscience* 30, no. 50 (2010): 17063–67.

24. R E Beaty et al., 'Creativity and the default network: A functional connectivity analysis of the creative brain at rest', *Neuropsychologia* 64 (2014): 92–98, doi:10.1016/j.neuropsychologia.2014.09.019; R E Beatty et al., 'Robust prediction of individual creative ability from brain functional connectivity', *Proceedings of the National Academy of Sciences* 115, no. 5 (30 January 2018): 1087–92.

25. B Draganski et al., 'Changes in grey matter induced by training', *Nature* 427 (22 January 2004): 6972.

26. J Boyke, J Driemeyer, C Gaser, C Büchel, and A May, 'Training-induced brain structure changes in the elderly', *Journal of Neuroscience* 28, no. 28 (9 July 2008): 7031–35.

27. N Charness et al., 'The role of deliberate practice in chess expertise', *Applied Cognitive Psychology* 19 (2005): 151–65.

28. W L Bryan and N Harter, 'Studies on the telegraphic language: The acquisition of a hierarchy of habits', *Psychological Review* 6, no. 4 (1899): 345–75.

29. K A Ericsson, R T Krampe, and C Tesch-Römer, 'The role of deliberate practice in the acquisition of expert performance', *Psychological Review* 100 (1993): 363–406.

30. F Gobet and M H Ereku, 'Checkmate to deliberate practice: The case of Magnus Carlsen', *Frontiers in Psychology* 5 (2014): 878, doi:10.3389/fpsyg.2014.00878.

31. K R Vickers et al., 'Attempted establishment of proficiency levels [. . .]', Surgical Endoscopy 21 (2007): 5–10; K R Vickers et al., 'Effects of pathologic stage on the learning curve for radical prostatectomy [. . .]', *European Urology* 53 (2008): 960–66; K R Vickers et al., 'The surgical learning curve laparoscopic radical prostatectomy: A retrospective cohort study', *The Lancet Oncology* 10 (2009): 475–80.

32. K A Ericsson, 'Deliberate practice and the acquisition and maintenance of expert performance in medicine and related domains', *Academic Medicine* 79 (2004): S70–80.

33. J Norcini et al., 'Certifying examination performance and patient outcomes following acute myocardial infarction', *Medical Education* 36 (2002): 853–59; J Norcini et al., 'Certification and specialization: Do they matter in the outcome of myocardial infarction?', *Academic Medicine* 75 (2000): 1193–98.

34. R H Wozniak, 'Introduction to Hermann Ebbinghaus (1885/1913)', *Classics in the History of Psychology* (1999), https://psychclassics.yorku.ca/Ebbinghaus/wozniak.htm; A G Bills, *General Experimental Psychology*, Longmans Psychology Series (New York: Longmans, Green and Co., 1934), 192–215.

## 4. What Kind of Learner Are You?

35. J. Biggs, 'Reflective thinking and school learning: An introduction to the theory and practice of metacognition', Item IO, *Set, Research Information for Teachers*, no. 2 (Wellington, NZ: NZCER, 1987): 10–11; J H Flavell, 'Metacognitive aspects of problem solving', in *The Nature of Intelligence*, ed. L B Resnick (Hillsdale, NJ: Lawrence Erlbaum, 1976), 231–35.

## 5. Success Does Not Equal Perfect

36. T Curran and A Hill, 'Perfectionism is increasing over time: A meta-analysis of birth cohort differences from 1989 to 2016', *Psychology Bulletin* 145, no. 4 (2019): 410–29; M M Smith et al., 'Why does socially prescribed perfectionism place people at risk for depression? A five-month, two-wave longitudinal study of the Perfectionism Social Disconnection Model', *Personality and Individual Differences* 134 (2018): 49–54.

37. R O Frost et al., 'The dimensions of perfectionism', *Cognitive Therapy and Research* 14 (1990): 449–68.

38. A M Burgess et al., 'Development and validation of the Frost Multidimensional Perfectionism Scale–Brief', *Journal of Psychoeducational Assessment* 34 (2016): 620–33; A M Stairs, G T Smith, T C Zapolski, J L Combs, and R E Settles, 'Clarifying the construct of perfectionism', *Assessment* 19, no. 2 (2012): 146–66, doi:10.1177/1073191111411663.

## 6. Passion for the Purpose

39. S Balon et al., 'Passion and personality: Is passionate behaviour a function of personality?', *European Review of Applied Psychology* 63 (2013): 59–65.

40. N Chamfort, Maximes et Pensées (Paris: Larousse, 1928).

41. Balon et al., 'Passion and personality'.

42. M E P Seligman and M Csikszentmihalyi, 'Positive psychology: An introduction', *American Psychologist* 55 (2000): 5–14.

43. R J Vallerand et al., 'Les passions de l'aˆme: On obsessive and harmonious passion', *Journal of Personality and Social Psychology* 85 (2003): 756–67.

44. R Vallerand, 'From motivation to passion: In search of the motivational processes involved in a meaningful life', *Canadian Psychology* 53 (2012): 42–52.

45. T Curran et al., 'The psychology of passion: A meta-analytical review of a decade of research on intrapersonal outcomes', *Motivation and Emotion* 39 (2015): 631–55, https://doi.org/10.1007/s11031-015-9503-0.

46. T Clohessy, E Whelan, and K Paradis, 'Does passion for physical activity spillover into performance at work? Examining the direct and indirect effects of passion and life satisfaction on organisational performance and innovativeness', *International Journal of Sport and Exercise Psychology* (22 May 2020): 1–2, doi:10.1080/1612197X.2020.1766537.

47. R J Vallerand, F L Rousseau, F M E Grouzet, A Dumais, and S Grenier, 'Passion in sport: A look at determinants and affective experiences', *Journal of Sport and Exercise Psychology* 28 (2006): 454–78.

48. F L Philippe, R J Vallerand, N Houlfort, G L Lavigne, and E G Donahue, 'Passion for an activity and quality of interpersonal relationships: The mediating role of emotions', *Journal of Personality and Social Psychology* 98, no. 6 (2010): 917–32.

49. A Bonneville-Roussy, G Lavigne and R J Vallerand, 'When passion leads to excellence: The case of musicians', *Psychology of Music* 39 (2011): 123–38.

50. G Mageau, R Vallerand, F Rousseau, C Ratelle, and P Provencher, 'Passion and gambling: Investigating the divergent affective and cognitive consequences of gambling', *Journal of Applied Social Psychology* 35 (2005): 100–118, doi:10.1111/j.1559- 1816.2005.tb02095.x.

51. K H Perttula and M S Cardon, 'Passion', in *The Oxford Handbook of Positive Organisational Scholarship*, ed. K S Cameron and G M Spreitzer (New York: Oxford University Press, 2011), 190–200.

52. C P Patel, S Thorgren, and J Wincent, 'Leadership, passion and performance: A study of job creation projects during the recession', *British Journal of Management* 26, no. 2 (2015): 211–24, doi:10.1111/1467-8551.12092.

53. M Ahearne, J Mathieu, and A Rapp, 'To empower or not to empower your sales force? An empirical examination of the influence of leadership empowerment behavior on customer satisfaction and performance', *Journal of Applied Psychology* 90 (2005): 945–55, doi:10.1037/0021-9010.90.5.945.

54. J Carpentier, G Mageau, and R J Vallerand, 'Ruminations and flow: Why do people with a more harmonious passion experience higher well-being?', *Journal of Happiness Studies* 13 (2012): 501–18, doi:10.1007/s10902-011-9276-4.

55. C F Ratelle, R J Vallerand, G A Mageau, F L Rousseau, and P Provencher, 'When passion leads to problematic outcomes: A look at gambling', *Journal of Gambling Studies* 20, no. 2 (2004): 105–19. doi:10.1023/B:JOGS.0000022304.96042.e6.

56. F Philippe, R J Vallerand, G Lavigne, 'Passion does make a difference in people's lives: A look at well-being in passionate and non-passionate individuals', *Applied Psychology: Health and Well-Being* 1 (2009): 3–22. doi:10.1111/j.1758-0854.2008.01003.x.

57. B Rip, S Fortin, and R Vallerand, 'The relationship between passion and injury in dance students', *Journal of Dance Medicine & Science* 10 (2006): 14–20.

58. Balon et al., 'Passion and personality'.

59. Balon et al., 'Passion and personality'.

## 7. Perseverance

60. Merriam-Webster Dictionary, s.v. 'perseverance', https://www.merriam-webster.com/dictionary/perseverance.

61. A L Duckworth et al., 'Grit: Perserverence and passion for long-term goals', *Journal of Personality and Psychology* 92 (2007): 1087–101.

62. M Credé, M C Tynan, and P D Harms, 'Much ado about grit: A meta-analytic synthesis of the grit literature', *Journal of Personality and Social Psychology* 113, no. 3 (2017): 492–511, https://doi.org/10.1037/pspp0000102.

63. Z Ivcevic and M Brackett, 'Predicting school success: Comparing conscientiousness, grit, and emotion regulation ability', *Journal of Research in Personality* 52 (2014): 29–36; K Rimfield et al., 'True grit and genetics: Predicting academic achievement from personality', *Journal of Personality and Social Psychology* 111 (2016): 780–89.

64. R Vallerand, 'From motivation to passion: In search of the motivational processes involved in a meaningful life', *Canadian Psychology* 53 (2012): 42–52.

65. A H Maslow, 'A theory of human motivation', *Psychology Review* 50 (1943): 370–96.

66. E L Deci, *Intrinsic Motivation* (New York: Plenum Press, 1975).

67. E L Deci, *The Psychology of Self-Determination* (Lexington, MA: DC Heath, 1980).

68. E L Deci, 'Effects of externally mediated rewards on intrinsic motivation', *Journal of Personality and Social Psychology* 18 (1971): 105–15, doi:10.1037/h0030644.

69. R de Charms, *Personal Causation: The Internal Affective Determinants of Behavior* (New York: Academic Press, 1968).

70. R W White, 'Motivation reconsidered: The concept of competence', *Psychological Review* 66 (1959): 297–333.

71. R J Vallerand, 'A hierarchical model of intrinsic and extrinsic motivation for sport and physical activity', in *Self-Determination Theory in Exercise and Sport*, ed. M S D Hagger and N L D Chatzisarantis (Champaign, IL: Human Kinetics, 2007), 255–79; R J Vallerand, B P O'Connor, and M Hamel, 'Motivation in later life: Theory and assessment', *International Journal of Aging and Human Development* 41 (1995): 221–38.

72. D Ariani, 'Personality and learning motivation', *European Journal of Business and Management* 5 (2013): 26–38.

73. O de Manzano et al., 'Individual differences in the proness to have flow experiences are linked to dopamine D2 receptor availability in the dorsal striatum', *Neuroimage* 67 (2013): 1–6.

74. S I di Domenic and R M Ryan, 'The emerging neuroscience of intrinsic motivation: A new frontier in self-determination research', *Frontiers in Human Neuroscience* 11 (2017): 145.

## 8. Conscientiousness

75. K L Jang, W J Livesley, and P A Vernon, 'Heritability of the Big Five personality dimensions and their facets: A twin study', *Journal of Personalized Medicine* 64, no. 3 (September 1996): 577–91, doi:10.1111/j.1467-6494.1996.tb00522.x. PMID: 8776880.

76. P T Costa and R R McCrae, *NEO Personality Inventory Professional Manual* (Odessa, FL: Psychological Assessment Resources, 1992).

77. K A Fleming, S J Heintzelman, and B D Bartholow, 'Specifying associations between conscientiousness and executive functioning: Mental set shifting, not prepotent response inhibition or working memory updating', *Journal of Personalized Medicine* 84, no. 3 (2016): 348–60, doi:10.1111/jopy.12163.

78. D Reiss, J S Eccles, and L Nielsen, 'Conscientiousness and public health: Synthesizing current research to promote healthy aging', *Developmental Psychology* 50, no. 5 (2014): 1303–14.

79. R D Goodwin and H S Friedman, 'Health status and the five-factor personality traits in a nationally representative sample', *Journal of Health Psychology*, 11, no. 5 (2006):, 643–54, doi:10.1177/1359105306066610.

80. B P Chapman, E van Wijngaarden, C L Seplaki, N Talbot, P Duberstein, and J Moynihan, 'Openness and conscientiousness predict 34-week patterns of Interleukin-6 in older persons', *Brain Behavior and Immunity* 25, no. 4 (2011): 667–73. doi:10.1016/j.bbi.2011.01.003.

81. M L Kern and H S Friedman, 'Personality and pathways of influence on physical health', *Social and Personality Psychology Compass* 5, no. 1 (2011): 76–87.

82. Andrew Steptoe et al., 'Conscientiousness, hair cortisol concentration, and health behaviour in older men and women', *Psychoneuroendocrinology* 86 (2017): 122–27.

83. D M Higgins et al., 'Prefrontal cognitive ability, intelligence, Big Five personality, and the prediction of advanced academic and workplace performance', *Journal of Personality and Social Psychology* 93, no. 2 (August 2007): 298–319; N M Dudley et al., 'A meta-analytic investigation of conscientiousness in the prediction of job performance: Examining the intercorrelations and the incremental validity of narrow traits', *Journal of Applied Psychology* 91 (2006): 40–57; T A Judge et al., 'The Big Five personality traits, general mental ability, and career success across the life span', *Personnel Psychology* 52 (1999): 621–52; E E Noftle and R W Robins, 'Personality predictors of academic outcomes: Big Five correlates of GPA and SAT scores', *Journal of Personality and Social Psychology* 93, no. 1 (July 2007): 116–30.

84. X Tran, 'Football scores on the Big Five personality factors across 50 States in the U.S.', *Journal of Sports Medicine & Doping Studies* 2 (2012): 117–21; R L Piedmont, D C Hill, and S Blanco, 'Predicting athletic performance using the five-factor model of personality', *Personality and Individual Differences* 27 (1997): 769–77.

85. M E Nia and M A Besharat, 'Comparison of athletes' personality characteristics in individual and team sports', *Procedia—Social and Behavioral Sciences* 5 (2010): 808–12.

86. M Komarraju and S J Karau, 'The relationship between the Big Five personality traits and academic motivation', *Personality and Individual Differences* 39 (2005): 557–67.

87. B Studer-Luethi et al., 'Influence of neuroticism and conscientiousness on working memory training outcome', *Personality and Individual Differences* (2012), doi:10.1016/j.paid.2012.02.012.

88. M P Wilmot and D Ones, 'A century of research on conscientiousness at work', *Proceedings of the National Academy of Sciences* 116, no. 46 (2019): 23004–10, doi:10.1073/pnas.1908430116.

89. J Stoeber et al., 'Perfectionism and the Big Five: Conscientiousness predicts longitudinal increases in self-oriented perfectionism', *Personality and Individual Differences* 47 (2009): 363–68.

90. B W Roberts et al., 'The power of personality: The comparative validity of personality traits, socioeconomic status, and cognitive ability for predicting important life outcomes', *Perspectives on Psychological Science* 2 (2007): 313–45; T Bogg and B W Roberts, 'The case for conscientiousness: Evidence and implications for a personality trait marker of health and longevity', *Annals of Behavioral Medicine* 45 (2013): 278–88.

91. C G DeYoung, L C Quilty, and J B Peterson, 'Between facets and domains: 10 aspects of the Big Five', *Journal of Personality and Social Psychology* 93 (2007): 880–96; 'The items in the Big Five aspects scale', International Personality Item Pool, https://ipip.ori.org/BFASKeys.htm#BFASConscientiousness.

92. O P John and S Srivastava, 'The Big-Five trait taxonomy: History, measurement, and theoretical perspectives', in *Handbook of Personality: Theory and Research*, vol. 2, ed. L A Pervin and O P John (New York: Guilford Press, 1999), 102–38.

93. K N Javaras, M Williams, and A R Baskin-Sommers, 'Psychological interventions potentially useful for increasing conscientiousness', *Personality Disorders: Theory, Research, and Treatment* 10 (2019): 13–24.

94. D T Neal, W Wood, J S Labrecque, and P Lally, 'How do habits guide behavior? Perceived and actual triggers of habits in daily life', *Journal of Experimental Social Psychology* 48 (2012): 492–98; W Wood and D T Neal, 'A new look at habits and the habit-goal interface', *Psychological Review* 114, no. 4 (October 2007): 843–63; P Lally, C H M van Jaarsveld, H W W Potts, and J Wardle, 'How are habits formed: Modelling habit formation in the real world', *European Journal of Social Psychology* 40, no. 6 (October 2010): 998–1009, doi:10.1002/ejsp.674.

95. Society for Personality and Social Psychology, 'How we form habits, change existing ones', *ScienceDaily*, 8 August 2014, www.sciencedaily.com/releases/2014/08/140808111931.htm.

96. P Lally et al., 'How are habits formed: Modelling habit formation in the real world', *European Journal Social Psychology* 40 (2010):998–1009.

97. N Kaushal amd R E Rhodes, 'Exercise habit formation in new gym members: A longitudinal study', *Journal of Behavioral Medicine* 38, no. 4 (August 2015): 652–63, doi:10.1007/s10865-015-9640-7.

## 9. Self-Efficacy

98. J E Maddux, 'The power of believing you can', in *The Oxford Handbook of Positive Psychology*, ed. S Lopez and C Snyder (Oxford: Oxford University Press, 2009).

99. A Bandura, *Self-Efficacy: The Exercise of Control* (New York: Freeman, 1997).

100. A Bandura, 'Social cognitive theory of self-regulation', *Organizational Behavior and Human Decision Processes* 50 (1991): 248–57.

101. Dr Seuss, *Oh the Places You'll Go* (New York: Random House, 1990).

102. W Piper, *The Little Engine that Could* (New York: Platt & Monk, 1930).

103. L Ross-Stewart and S E Short, 'The frequency and perceived effectiveness of images used to build, maintain, and regain confidence', *Journal of Applied Sport Psychology* 21, no. S1 (2009):S34–S47.

104. Northern Ireland Statistics and Research Agency, 'Self-efficacy, locus of control and life satisfaction', https://www.nisra.gov.uk/statistics/people-places-and-culture/self-efficacy-locus-control-and-life-satisfaction.

105. J E Maddux and R W Rogers, 'Protection motivation and self-efficacy: A revised theory of fear appeals and attitude change', *Journal of Experimental Social Psychology* 19 (1983): 469–79; R W Rogers and S Prentice-Dunn, 'Protection motivation theory', in *Handbook of Health Behavior Research 1: Personal and Social Determinants*, ed. D Gochman (New York: Plenum, 1997), 113–32; V J Strecher, V L Champion, and I M Rosenstock, 'The health belief model and health behavior', in *Handbook of Health Behavior Research*: 71–91; I Ajzen, *Attitudes, Personality, and Behavior* (Chicago: Dorsey Press, 1988).

106. A O'Leary and S Brown, 'Self-efficacy and the physiological stress response', in *Self-Efficacy, Adaptation, and Adjustment: Theory, Research, and Application*, ed. J E Maddux (New York: Plenum, 1995), 227–48.

107. J E Maddux, L Brawley, and A Boykin, 'Self-efficacy and healthy decision-making: Protection, promotion, and detection', in *Self-Efficacy, Adaptation, and Adjustment: Theory, Research, and Application*, ed. J E Maddux (New York: Plenum, 1995), 173–202.

108. R F Oman and A C King, 'Predicting the adoption and maintenance of exercise participation using self-efficacy and previous exercise participation rates', *American Journal of Health Promotion* 12, no. 3 (January-February 1998): 154–61.

109. J A Linde, A J Rothman, A S Baldwin, and R W Jeffery, 'The impact of self-efficacy on behavior change and weight change among overweight participants in a weight loss trial', *Health Psychology* 25, no. 3 (May 2006): 282–91.

110. J E Maddux and L J Meier, 'Self-efficacy and depression', in *Self-Efficacy, Adaptation, and Adjustment: Theory, Research, and Application* (New York: Plenum, 1995), 143–69.

111. A D Stajkovic and F Luthans, 'Self-efficacy and work-related performance: A meta-analysis', *Psychological Bulletin* 124 (1998): 240–61.

112. R Wood et al., 'Mechanisms governing organizational performance in complex decision-making', *Organizational Behavior and Human Decision Processes* 46 (1990): 181–201.

113. T Mitchell et al., 'Predicting self-efficacy and performance during skill acquisition', *Journal of Applied Psychology* 79 (1994): 506–17.

114. M E Gist, 'Self-efficacy: Implications for organizational behavior and human resource management', *Academic Management Review* 12 (1987): 472–85; K Jordan and R Carden, 'Self-efficacy and gender in STEM majors,' *Modern Psychological Studies* 22, no. 2, art. 8 (2017).

115. S Stumpf et al., 'Self-efficacy expectations and coping with career-related events', *Journal of Vocational Behavior* 31 (1987): 91–108.

116. T Hill, N D Smith, and M F Mann, 'Role of efficacy expectations in predicting the decision to use advanced technologies: The case of computers', *Journal of Applied Psychology* 72, no. 2 (1987): 307–13.

117. A M Saks, 'Longitudinal field investigation of the moderating and mediating effects of self-efficacy on the relationship between training and newcomer adjustment', *Journal of Applied Psychology* 80, no. 2 (1995): 211–25.

118. D Eden and Y Zuk, 'Seasickness as a self-fulfilling prophecy: Raising self-efficacy to boost performance at sea', *Journal of Applied Psychology* 80 (1995): 628–35.

119. A Abele and D Spurk, 'The longitudinal impact of self-efficacy and career goals on objective and subjective career success', *Journal of Vocational Behaviour* (2009): 53–62.

120. A Stajkovic and F Luthans, 'Self-efficacy and work-related performance: A meta-analysis, *Psychological Bulletin* 124 (1998): 240–61, doi:10.1037/0033-2909.124.2.240.

121. E Litzler et al., 'Breaking it down: Engineering student STEM confidence at the intersection of race/ethnicity and gender', *Research in Higher Education* 55 (2014): 810–32.

122. E A Locke, E Zubritzky, E Cousins, and P Bobko, 'Effect of previously assigned goals on self-set goals and performance', *Journal of Applied Psychology* 69 (1984): 694–99; D H Schunk, 'Enhancing self-efficacy and achievement through rewards and goals: Motivational and informational effects', *Journal of Educational Research* 78 (1984): 29–34.

123. C Huang, 'Gender differences in academic self-efficacy: A meta-analysis', *European Journal of Psychology of Education* 28 (2013).

124. C Hill et al., Why So Few? Women in Science, Technology, Engineering and Mathematics (Washington, DC: AAUW, 2010).

125. J J Siegfried, 'Male-female differences in economic education: A survey', *Journal of Economic Education* 10 (1979): 1–11; M A Ferber et al., 'Gender differences in economic knowledge: A re-evaluation of the evidence', *Journal of Economic Education* 14 (1983): 24–37; L Opstad and L Fallan, 'Student performance in principles of economics: The importance of gender and personality', *International Review of Economics Education* 9 (2010): 76–92; B Anderson, H Benjamin, and M A Fuss, 'The determinants of success in university introductory economics courses', *Journal of Economic Education* 25 (1994): 99–119.

126. A Bandura, 'Social cognitive theory', in *Six Theories of Child Development*, ed. R Vasta, vol. 6 of *Annals of Child Development* (London: Jessica Kingsley, 1989), 1–60.

127. S Moritz, D Feltz, K Fahrbach, and D Mack, 'The relation of self-efficacy measures to sport performance: A meta-analytic review', *Research Quarterly for Exercise and Sport* 71 (2000): 280–94; V H Sklett et al. 'Self-efficacy, flow, affect, worry and performance in elite World Cup ski jumping', *Frontiers in Psychology* 9 (17 July 2018): 1215, doi:10.3389/fpsyg.2018.01215. PMID: 30065687; PMCID: PMC6057433; J Barling and M Abel, 'Self-efficacy beliefs and tennis performance', *Cognitive Therapy and Research* 7 (1983): 265–72 (1983); D Feltz and C Lirgg, 'Self-efficacy beliefs of athletes, teams, and coaches', *Handbook of Sports Psychology* 2 (2001): 340–61; R L Woolfolk, S M Murphy, D Gottesfeld, and D Aitken, 'Effects of mental rehearsal of task motor activity and mental depiction of task outcome on motor skill performance', *Journal of Sport Psychology* 7, no. 2 (1985): 191–97; S K Wurtele, 'Self-efficacy and athletic performance: a review', *Journal of Social and Clinical Psychology* 4 (1986): 290–301.

128. T M Okwumabua, 'Psychological and physical contributions to marathon performance: An exploratory investigation', *Journal of Sport Behavior* 8 (1985): 163–71; I Heazlewood and S Burke, 'Self-efficacy and its relationship to selected sport psychological constructs in the prediction of performance in ironman triathlon', *Journal of Human Sport and Exercise* 6, no. 2 (2011): 328–50.

129. Wurtele, 'Self-efficacy and athletic performance'.

130. J C Hutchinson, T Sherman, N Martinovic, and G Tenenbaum, 'The effect of manipulated self-efficacy on perceived and sustained effort', *Journal of Applied Sport Psychology* 20, no. 4 (2008): 457–72.

131. G Tenenbaum et al., 'Coping with physical exertion and negative feedback under competitive and self-standard conditions', *Journal of Applied Social Psychology* 31, no. 8 (2001): 1582–626.

132. G Chen and P D Bliese, 'The role of different levels of leadership in predicting self- and collective efficacy: Evidence for discontinuity', *Journal of Applied Psychology* 87 (2002): 549–56.

133. T Rigotti et al., 'Career-related self-efficacy, its antecedents and relationship to subjective career success in a cross-lagged panel study', *International Journal of Human Resource Management* 31, no. 20 (2020): 2645–72.

## 10. Self-Awareness

134. F Jabr, 'Does self-awareness require a complex brain?', Scientific American (22 August 2012), https://blogs.scientificamerican.com/brainwaves/does-self-awareness-require-a-complex-brain/#:~:text=Scientists%20differ%20on%20the%20difference,that%20one%20is%20aware%20of.

135. C Philippi, J S Feinstein, S S Khalsa, A Damasio, D Tranel, G Landini, K Williford, and D Rudrauf, 'Preserved self-awareness following extensive bilateral brain damage to the insula, anterior cingulate, and medial prefrontal cortices', *PLoS One* (22 August 2012).

136. T Eurich, 'What self-awareness really is (and how to cultivate it)', *Harvard Business Review* (4 January 2018).

137. P J Silvia and M O'Brien, 'Self-awareness and constructive functioning: Revisiting "the human dilemma"', *Journal of Social and Clinical Psychology* 23 (2004): 475–89; A Sutton et al., 'A longitudinal, mixed method evaluation of self-awareness training in the workplace', *European Journal of Training and Development* 39 (2015): 610–27; A H Church, 'Managerial self-awareness in high performing individuals in organisations', *Journal of Applied Psychology* 82 (1997): 281–92.

138. J Kruger and D Dunning, 'Unskilled and unaware of it: How difficulties in recognizing one's own incompetence lead to inflated self-assessments', *Journal of Personality and Social Psychology* 77, no. 6 (1999): 1121–34.

139. J Ehrlinger et al., 'Why the unskilled are unaware: Further explorations of (absent) self-insight among the incompetent', *Organizational Behavior and Human Decision Processes* 105, no. 1 (2008): 98–121.

140. C Lee, 'Revisiting why incompetents think they're awesome', *Ars Technica* (4 November 2016), https://arstechnica.com/science/2016/11/revisiting-why-incompetents-think-theyre-awesome.

141. C G Jung, *Memories, Dreams, Reflections* (1961; repr., New York: Vintage Books, 1989).

142. 'MTBI Basics', Myers Briggs Foundation, https://www.myersbriggs.org/my-mbti-personality-type/mbti-basics.

143. R Eveleth, 'The Myers Briggs Personality Test is pretty much meaningless', *Smithsonian Magazine* (26 March 2013), https://www.smithsonianmag.com/smart-news/the-myers-briggs-personality-test-is-pretty-much-meaningless-9359770.

144. B R Forer, 'The fallacy of personal validation: A classroom demonstration of gullibility', *Journal of Abnormal and Social Psychology* 44, no. 1 (1949): 118–23.

145. J Luft and H Ingham, 'The Johari window, a graphic model of interpersonal awareness' (proceedings of the Western Training Laboratory in Group Development, University of California, Los Angeles, 1955).

146. G Di Stefano et al., 'Making experience count: The role of reflection in individual learning' (working paper 14-093, Harvard Business School, 2014); J M Jachimowicz et al., 'Commuting as role transitions: How trait self-control and work related prospection offset negative effects of lengthy commutes' (working paper 16-077, Harvard Business School, 2016).

## 11. Vitality

147. World Health Organization, 'Constitution', https://www.who.int/about/who-we-are/constitution.

148. C Dweck *Mindset: How You Can Fulfil Your Potential* (London: Constable & Robinson, 2012).

149. Dweck, *Mindset*.

150. Dweck, *Mindset*.

151. H Selye, 'A syndrome produced by diverse nocuous agents', *Nature* 138 (4 July 4 1936): 32; reprinted in the *Journal of Neuropsychiatry* 10 (1998): 230–31.

152. V R LeBlanc, 'The effects of acute stress on performance: Implications for health professions education', *Academy of Medicine* 84, no. 10 Suppl (2009): S25–S33.

153. M Wheelock et al., 'Prefrontal cortex activity is associated with biobehavioral components of the stress response', *Frontiers in Human Neuroscience* (17 November 2016).

154. M Williams and D Pennyman, *Mindfulness: A Practical Guide to Finding Peace in a Frantic World* (London: Paitkus, 2011).

155. J Kabat-Zinn et al., 'Effectiveness of a meditation-based stress reduction program in the treatment of anxiety disorders', *American Journal of Psychiatry* 149, no. 7 (1992): 936–43. https://doi.org/10.1176/ajp.149.7.936 PMID: 1609875; J Miller, K Fletcher, and J Kabat-Zinn, 'Three-year follow-up and clinical implications of a mindfulness- based stress reduction intervention in the treatment of anxiety disorders', *General Hospital Psychiatry* 17 (1995): 192–200, PMID: 7649463; D K Reibel, J M Greeson, G C Brainard, and S Rosenzweig, 'Mindfulness-based stress reduction and health-related quality of life in a heterogeneous patient population', *General Hospital Psychiatry* 23 (2001): 183–92. PMID: 11543844.

156. M C Davis, A J Zautra, L D Wolf, H Tennen, and E W Yeung, 'Mindfulness and cognitive-behavioral interventions for chronic pain: Differential effects on daily pain reactivity and stress reactivity', *Journal of Consulting and Clinical Psychology* 83, no. 1 (2015): 24–35.

157. D S Black and G M Slavich, 'Mindfulness meditation and the immune system: A systematic review of randomized controller trials', *Annals of the New York Academy of Sciences* 1373 (2016): 13–24, doi.org/10.1111/nyas.12998 PMID: 26799456.

158. M Goyal et al., 'Meditation programs for psychological stress and well-being: A systematic review and meta-analysis', *JAMA Internal Medicine* 174 (2014): 357–68.

159. M Janssen et al., 'Effects of mindfulness-based stress reduction on employees' mental health: A systematic review', *PLoS One* 13, no. 1 (2018): e01911332.

160. B Holzel et al., 'Mindfulness practice leads to increases in regional brain gray matter density', *Psychiatry Research* 191, no. 1 (2011): 36–43.

161. J Kabat-Zinn, *Full Catastrophe Living: Using the Wisdom of Your Body and Mind to Face Stress, Pain, and Illness* (New York: Delacorte, 1990).

162. Sheldon Cohen, 'Perceived Stress Scale', Mind Garden, 1984, https://www.mindgarden.com/documents/PerceivedStressScale.pdf.

163. J Nakamura and M Csikszentmihalyi, 'Flow Theory and Research', in *The Oxford Handbook of Positive Psychology*, ed. C R Snyder, E Wright, and S Lopez (Oxford: Oxford University Press, 2011), 195–206.

## 12. Chronobiology

164. A Lee and J C Galvez, 'Jet lag in athletes', *Sports Health* 4, no. 3 (2012): 211–16, https://www.ncbi.nlm.nih.gov/pmc/articles/PMC3435929.

165. J F Duffy and C A Czeisler, 'Age-related change in the relationship between circadian period, circadian phase, and diurnal preference in humans', *Neuroscience Letters* 318 (2002): 117–20; D Fischer, D A Lombardi, H Marucci-wellman, and T Roenneberg, 'Chronotypes in the US—influence of age and sex', *PLoS One* 12 (2017): e0178782; K V Allebrandt et al., 'Chronotype and sleep duration: The influence of season of assessment', *Chronobiology International* 31 (2014): 731–740; S Jones et al., 'Genome-wide association analyses of chronotype in 697,828 individuals provides insights into circadian rhythms', *Nature Communications* 10, no. 343 (2019), doi:10.1038/s41467-018-08259-7.

166. C Randler, C Faßl, and N Kalb, 'From lark to owl: Developmental changes in morningness-eveningness from new-borns to early adulthood.', *Scientific Reports* 7, no. 45874 (2017).

167. M Wieth and R Zacks, 'Time of day effects on problem solving: When the non-optimal is optimal', *Thinking and Reasoning* 17 (2011): 387–401

168. Jones et al., 'Genome-wide association analyses of chronotype'; F Patterson et al., 'Interactive effects of sleep duration and morning/evening preference on cardiovascular risk factors', *European Journal of Public Health* 28 (2018): 155–61; I Merikanto et al., 'Associations of chronotype and sleep with cardiovascular diseases and type 2 diabetes', *Chronobiology International* 30 (2013): 470–77; R Levandovski et al., 'Depression scores associate with chronotype and social jetlag in a rural population', *Chronobiology International* 28 (2011): 771–78.

169. E L Rossi, *The Twenty Minute Break: Reduce Stress, Maximize Performance, Improve Health and Emotional Well-Being Using the New Science of Ultradian Rhythms* (Phoenix, AZ: Zeig, Tucker & Co, 2000).

170. S Kim et al., 'Daily micro-breaks and job performance: General work engagement as a cross-level moderator', *Journal of Applied Psychology* 103, no. 7 (2018):772–86.

## 13. Fitness

171. N Owen et al., 'Sedentary behavior: Emerging evidence for a new health risk', *Mayo Clinic Proceedings* 85, no. 12 (2010):1138–41.

172. D W Dunstan and N Owen, 'New exercise prescription: Don't just sit there: Stand up and move more, more often', *Archives of Internal Medicine* 172, no. 6 (2012): 500–501; A V Patel, L Bernstein, A Deka, H S Feigelson, P T Campbell, S M Gapstur, G A Colditz, and M J Thun, 'Leisure time spent sitting in relation to total mortality in a prospective cohort of US adults', *American Journal of Epidemiology* 172, no. 4 (15 August 2010):419–29; M J Wheeler et al., 'Sedentary behavior as a risk factor for cognitive decline? A focus on the influence of glycemic control in brain health', *Alzheimer's and Dementia: Translational Research and Clinical Interventions* 3 (2017): 291–300. N Owen et al., 'Sedentary behavior'; D Thivel, A Tremblay, P M Genin, S Panahi, D Rivière, and M Duclos, 'Physical activity, inactivity, and sedentary behaviors: Definitions and implications in occupational health', *Frontiers in Public Health* 6 (2018): 288, doi:10.3389/fpubh.2018.00288. D W Dunstan, E L M Barr, G N Healy, et al. 'Television viewing time and mortality: The AusDiab study', *Circulation* 121, no. 3 (2010):384–91. P T Katzmarzyk, T S Church, C L Craig, and C Bouchard, 'Sitting time and mortality from all causes, cardiovascular disease, and cancer', *Medicine and Science in Sports and Exercise* 41, no. 5 (2009):998–1005.

173. Wheeler et al., 'Sedentary behavior as a risk factor for cognitive decline?'

174. Wheeler et al., 'Sedentary behavior as a risk factor for cognitive decline?'

175. 'Physical Activity Recommendations for Different Age Groups', Centers for Disease Control and Prevention, last reviewed 17 September 2020, https://www.cdc.gov/physicalactivity/basics/age-chart.html.

176. The source for tables 13.2, 13.3, and 13.4 is American College of Sports Medicine, *ACSM's Guidelines for Exercise Testing and Prescription*, 10th rev. ed. (Philadelphia: Lippincott Williams and Wilkins, 2017).

177. A Mika et al., 'Comparison of recovery strategies on muscle performance after fatiguing exercise', *American Journal of Physical Medicine and Rehabilitation* 86, no. 6 (2007): 474–81; A Barnett, 'Using recovery modalities between training sessions in elite athletes', *Sports Medicine* 36 (2006): 781–96; J C Andersen, 'Stretching before and after exercise: Effect on muscle soreness and injury risk', *Journal of Athletic Training* 40 (2005): 218–20; I Shrier, 'Does stretching improve performance? A systematic and critical review of the literature', *Clinical Journal of Sports Medicine* 14 (2004): 267–73; Q A Soltow, J L Betters, J E Sellman, et al., 'Ibroprofen inhibits skeletal muscle hypertrophy in rats', *Medicine and Science in Sports and Exercise* 38 (2006): 840–46; T A Trappe, F White, C P Lambert, et al. 'Effect of ibuprofen and acetaminophen on postexercise muscle protein synthesis', *American Journal of Physiology-Endocrinology and Metabolism* 282 (2002): E551–56.

178. S Herman et al., 'Four-week dynamic stretching warm-up intervention elicits longer-term performance benefits', *Journal of Strength and Conditioning Research* 22 (2008): 1286–97; F Ingjer and S B StrØmme, 'Effects of active, passive or no warm-up on the physiological response to heavy exercise', *European Journal of Applied Physiology* 40 (1979): 273–82; C P Busuttil and R O Ruhling, 'Warm-up and circulo-respiratory adaptations', *Journal of Sports Medicine* 17 (1977): 69–74; E R Elbel and W J Mikols, 'The effects of passive or active warm-up upon certain physiological measures', *Internationale Zeitschrift für Angewandte Physiologie* 31 (1972): 41–52.

179. For further information, see P Han et al., 'Clinical evidence of exercise benefits for stroke', *Advances in Experimental Medicine and Biology* 1000 (2017): 131–51; R W Motl and B M Sandroff, 'Benefits of exercise training in multiple sclerosis', *Current Neurology and Neuroscience Reports* 15, no. 9 (2015): 62; C Fiuza-Luces et al., 'Exercise benefits in cardiovascular disease: Beyond attenuation of traditional risk factors', *Nature Reviews Cardiology* 15, no. 12 (December 2018): 731–43; N L Stout et al., 'A systematic review of exercise systematic reviews in the cancer literature (2005–2017)', *Physical Medicine and Rehabilitation* 9 (17 September 2017): S347–84; B Stubbs et al., 'An examination of the anxiolytic effects of exercise for people with anxiety and stress-related disorders: A meta-analysis', *Psychiatry Research* 249 (March 2017): 102–8; T Archer et al., 'Effects of physical exercise on depressive symptoms and biomarkers in depression', *CNS Neurological Disorders—Drug Targets* 13, no. 10 (2014):1640–53; J E Lang, 'The impact of exercise on asthma', *Current Opinion in Allergy and Clinical Immunology* 19, no. 2 (April 2019):118–25; J P Kirwan et al., 'The essential role of exercise in the management of type 2 diabetes', *Cleveland Clinic Journal of Medicine* 84, no. 7 Suppl. 1 (July 2017): S15–S21.

180. American College of Sports Medicine, *ACSM's Guidelines for Exercise Testing and Prescription.*

181. J Laforgia, R T Withers, and C J Gore, 'Effects of exercise intensity and duration on the excess post-exercise oxygen consumption', *Journal of Sports Sciences* 24, no. 12 (2006): 1247–64.

182. Z Wang, Z Ying, A Bosy-Westphal, et al., 'Specific metabolic rates of major organs and tissues across adulthood: Evaluation by mechanistic model of resting energy expenditure', *American Journal of Clinical Nutrition* 92, no. 6 (2010): 1369–77.

183. L Sylow and E A Richter, 'Current advances in our understanding of exercise as medicine in metabolic disease', *Current Opinion in Physiology* 12 (December 2019): 12–19.

184. L B Borghouts and H A Keizer, 'Exercise and insulin sensitivity: A review', International *Journal of Sports Medicine* 21, no. 1 (January 2000): 1–12; L Sylow and E A Richter, 'Current advances in our understanding of exercise as medicine in metabolic disease', *Current Opinion in Physiology* 12 (December 2019): 12–19.

185. Sylow and Richter, 'Current advances in our understanding of exercise as medicine in metabolic disease'.

186. M C Pensel, M Daamen, L Scheef, et al., 'Executive control processes are associated with individual fitness outcomes following regular exercise training: Blood lactate profile curves and neuroimaging findings', *Scientific Reports 8*, no. 4893 (2018); M W Voss et al., 'Bridging animal and human models of exercise-induced brain plasticity', *Trends in Cognitive Sciences* 17, no. 10 (2013): 525–44; A F Kramer, K I Erickson, and S J Colcombe, 'Exercise, cognition, and the aging brain', *Journal of Applied Physiology* (1985) 101, no. 4 (2006): 1237–42; E Duzel, H van Praag, and M Sendtner, 'Can physical exercise in old age improve memory and hippocampal function?' *Brain* 139, pt. 3 (2016): 662–73; C Vivar, 'Adult hippocampal neurogenesis, aging and neurodegenerative diseases: Possible strategies to prevent cognitive impairment', *Current Topics in Medicinal Chemistry* 15, no. 21 (2015): 2175–92; C Vivar, M C Potter, and H van Praag, 'All about running: Synaptic plasticity, growth factors and adult hippocampal neurogenesis', *Current Topics in Behavioral Neurosciences* 15 (2013): 189–210; H van Praag, 'Neurogenesis and exercise: Past and future directions', *Neuromolecular Medicine* 10, no. 2 (2008): 128–40; Y K Chang et al., 'The effects of acute exercise on cognitive performance: A meta-analysis', *Brain Research* 1453 (2012): 87–101.

187. J C Basso and W A Suzuki, 'The effects of acute exercise on mood, cognition, neurophysiology, and neurochemical pathways: A review', *Brain Plasticity* 2, no. 2 (2017): 127–52.

188. Chang et al., 'The effects of acute exercise on cognitive performance'.

189. Y K Chang and J L Etnier, 'Exploring the dose-response relationship between resistance exercise intensity and cognitive function', *Journal of Sport and Exercise Psychology* 31, no. 5 (2009): 640–56; P D Loprinzi and C J Kane, 'Exercise and cognitive function: A randomized controlled trial examining acute exercise and free-living physical activity and sedentary effects', *Mayo Clinic Proceedings* 90, no. 4 (2015): 450–60; C J Brush et al., 'Dose-response and time course effects of acute resistance exercise on executive function', *Journal of Sport and Exercise Psychology* (2016): 1–35; M Oberste et al., 'Do reported effects of acute aerobic exercise on subsequent higher cognitive performances remain if tested against an instructed self-myofascial release training control group? A randomized controlled trial', *PLoS One* 11, no. 12 (2016): e0167818; Y K Chang et al., 'Dose-response effect of acute resistance exercise on Tower of London in middle-aged adults', *Journal of Sport and Exercise Psychology* 33, no. 6 (2011): 866–83.

190. F Chen et al., 'Effects of exercise modes on neural processing of working memory in late middle-aged adults: An fMRI study', *Frontiers in Aging Neuroscience* 11 (2019): 224ff.

191. Baso and Suzuki, 'The effects of acute exercise on mood, cognition, neurophysiology, and neurochemical pathways'.

192. Basso and Suzuki, 'The effects of acute exercise on mood, cognition, neurophysiology, and neurochemical pathways'; R E Thayer et al., 'Self-regulation of mood: Strategies for changing a bad mood, raising energy, and reducing tension', *Journal of Personality and Social Psychology* 67 (1994): 910–25.

193. P R Crocker and C Grozelle, 'Reducing induced state anxiety: Effects of acute aerobic exercise and autogenic relaxation', *Journal of Sports Medicine and Physical Fitness* 31, no. 2 (1991): 277–82; M Hamer, A Taylor, and A Steptoe, 'The effect of acute aerobic exercise on stress related blood pressure responses: A systematic review and meta-analysis', *Biological Psychology* 71, no. 2 (2006): 183–90; K A Brownley et al., 'Sympathoadrenergic mechanisms in reduced hemodynamic stress responses after exercise', *Medicine and Science in Sports and Exercise* 35, no. 6 (2003): 978–86.

194. J B Bartholomew, D Morrison, and J T Ciccolo, 'Effects of acute exercise on mood and well-being in patients with major depressive disorder', *Medicine and Science in Sports and Exercise* 37, no. 12 (2005): 2032–37; J Knapen et al., 'State anxiety and subjective well-being responses to acute bouts of aerobic exercise in patients with depressive and anxiety disorders', *British Journal of Sports Medicine* 43, no. 10 (2009): 756–59; J Heggelund et al., 'High aerobic intensity training and psychological states in patients with depression or schizophrenia', *Frontiers in Psychiatry* 5 (2014): 148; S J Petruzzello et al., 'A meta-analysis on the anxiety-reducing effects of acute and chronic exercise: Outcomes and mechanisms', *Sports Medicine* 11, no. 3 (1991): 143–82.

195. W Teo et al., 'Circadian rhythms in exercise performance: Implications for hormonal and muscular adaptation', *Journal of Sports Science and Medicine* 10, no. 4 (2011): 600–606.

196. N Souissi et al., Effects of regular training at the same time of day on diurnal fluctuations in muscular performance', *Journal of Sport Sciences* 20 (2002): 929–37; M Giacomoni et al., 'Effects of the time of day on repeated all-out cycle performance and short-term recovery patterns', *International Journal of Sports Medicine* 27 (2006): 468–74; N Bessot et al., 'The influence of circadian rhythm on muscle activity and efficient force production during cycling at different pedal rates', *Journal of Electromyography and Kinesiology* 17, no. 2 (April 2007):176–83; T Bernard et al. 'Time-of-day effects in maximal anaerobic leg exercise', *European Journal of Applied Physiology and Occupational Physiology* 77 (1998): 133–38; Teo et al., 'Circadian rhythms in exercise performance'.

197. M G Arnett, 'The effect of a morning and afternoon practice schedule on morning and afternoon swim performance', *Journal of Strength and Conditioning Research* 15 (February 2001): 127–31; L Martin and K Thompson, 'Reproducibility of diurnal variation in sub-maximal swimming', *International Journal of Sports Medicine* 21 (2000): 387–92; M G Arnett, 'Effects of prolonged and reduced warm-ups on diurnal variation in body temperature and swim performance', *Journal of Strength and Conditioning Research* 16 (2002): 256–61.

198. W Teo, M J Newton, and M R McGuigan, 'Circadian rhythms in exercise performance: Implications for hormonal and muscular adaptation', *Journal of Sports Science and Medicine* 10, no. 4 (2011):600–606.

199. Teo et al., 'Circadian rhythms in exercise performance'.

200. T Reilly et al., 'Diurnal variation in temperature, mental and physical performance, and tasks specifically related to football (soccer)', *Chronobiol International* 24, no. 3 (2007):507–19; G Atkinson and L Speirs, 'Diurnal variation in tennis service', *Perceptual and Motor Skills* 86 (1998): 1335–38; B Edwards et al., 'Can cycling performance in an early morning, laboratory-based cycle time-trial be improved by morning exercise the day before?', *International Journal of Sports Medicine* 26 (2005): 651–56.

201. F Brown et al., 'Collegiate rowing crew performance varies by morningness-eveningness', *Journal of Strength and Conditioning Research* 22 (2008): 1894–1900; D Hill et al., 'Diurnal variations in responses to exercise of "morning types" and "evening types"', *Journal of Sports Medicine and Physical Fitness* 28, no. 3 (September 1988): 213–19.

202. S D Youngstedt, J A Elliott, and D F Kripke, 'Human circadian phase-response curves for exercise', *Journal of Physiology* 597, no. 8 (2019): 2253–68.

203. J M Harrington, 'Health effects of shift work and extended hours of work', *Occupational and Environmental Medicine* 58 (2001): 68–72; A Knutsson, 'Health disorders of shift workers', *Occupational Medicine* (London) 53, no. 2 (March 2003): 103–8; J-A Lie et al., 'Night work and breast cancer risk among Norwegian nurses: Assessment by different exposure metrics', *American Journal of Epidemiology* 173 (2011): 1272–79; S Asaoka et al., 'Factors associated with shift work disorder in nurses working with rapid-rotation schedules in Japan: The nurses' sleep health project', *Chronobiology International* 30 (2013): 628–36; H Boggild and A Knutson, 'Shiftwork, risk factors and cardiovascular disease', *Scandinavian Journal of Work, Environment, and Health* 25 (1999): 85–99; S Folkard et al., 'Shiftwork: Safety, sleepiness and sleep', *Industrial Health* 43 (2005): 20–23.

204. Youngstedt, Elliott, and Kripke, 'Human circadian phase-response curves for exercise'.

205. Youngstedt, Elliott, and Kripke, 'Human circadian phase-response curves for exercise'; O Buxton et al., 'Exercise elicits phase shifts and acute alterations of melatonin that vary with circadian phase', *American Journal of Physiology—Regulatory, Integrative and Comparative Physiology* 284 (2003): R714–24; O Buxton et al., 'Roles of intensity and duration of nocturnal exercise in causing phase delays of human circadian rhythms', *American Journal of Physiology—Endocrinology and Metabolism* 273 (1997): E536–42.

206. E K Baehr, L F Fogg, and C I Eastman, 'Intermittent bright light and exercise to entrain human circadian rhythms to night work', *American Journal of Physiology* 277, no. 6 (December 1999): R1598–604.

207. L A Tucker, 'Physical activity and telomere length in U.S. men and women: An NHANES investigation', *Preventive Medicine* 100 (2017): 145, doi: 10.1016/j.ypmed.2017.04.027.

208. The source for tables 13.9 and 13.10 is American College of Sports Medicine, *ACSM's Guidelines for Exercise Testing and Prescription*.

## 14. Fitness in the High Performance Athlete

209. I I Ahmetov, O L Vinogradova, and A G Williams, 'Gene polymorphisms and fiber-type composition of human skeletal muscle', *International Journal of Sports Nutrition and Exercise Metabolism* 22, no. 4 (August 2012): 292–303.

210. C H Wyndham and N B Strydom, 'The danger of an inadequate water intake during marathon running', *South African Medical Journal* 43 (1969): 893–96.

211. D Lorenz et al., 'What performance characteristics determine elite versus nonelite athletes in the same sport?', *Sports Health* 5 (2013): 542–47.

212. Guinness World Records, 'Fastest badminton hit in competition (male)', https://www.guinnessworldrecords.com/world-records/fastest-badminton-hit-in-competition-(male).

213. D T Mann, A M Williams, P Ward, and C M Janelle, 'Perceptual-cognitive expertise in sport: A meta-analysis', *Journal of Sport and Exercise Psychology* 29 (2007): 457–78; B T Barrett, A G Cruickshank, J C Flavell, et al., 'Faster visual reaction times in elite athletes are not linked to better gaze stability', *Scientific Reports* 10 (2020): 13216.

214. C H Ooi et al., 'Physiological characteristics of elite and sub-elite badminton players', *Journal of Sports Science* 27, no. 14 (December 2009): 1591–99.

## 15. Nutrition for Us All

215. International Food Information Council (IFIC) Foundation, "Americans find doing their own taxes simpler than improving diet and health', *ScienceDaily* (23 May 2012), www.sciencedaily.com/releases/2012/05/120523145655.htm.

216. Centers for Disease Control and Prevention, 'About adult BMI', https://www.cdc.gov/healthyweight/assessing/bmi/adult_bmi/index.html.

217. C J Henry, 'Basal metabolic rate studies in humans: Measurement and development of new equations', *Public Health Nutrition* 8, no. 7A (October 2005): 1133–52.

218. J A Harris and F G Benedict, 'A Biometric Study of Human Basal Metabolism', *Proceedings of the National Academy of Sciences of the United States of America* 4, no. 12 (1918): 370–73.

219. K Westerterp et al., 'Energy expenditure and physical activity in subjects consuming full- or reduced-fat diets', *British Journal of Nutrition* 76 (1996): 785–95.

220. Z Wang et al., 'Evaluation of specific metabolic rates of major organs and tissues: Comparison between men and women', *American Journal of Human Biology* 23, no. 3 (2011): 333–38.

221. M Klok et al., 'The role of leptin and ghrelin in the regulation of food intake and body weight in humans: A review', *Obesity Reviews* 8, no. 1 (January 2007): 21–34.

222. C Mantzoros et al., 'A longitudinal assessment of hormonal and physical alterations during normal puberty in boys. V. Rising leptin levels may signal the onset of puberty', *Journal of Clinical Endocrinology and Metabolism* 82 (1997) 1066–70; G Lord et al., 'Leptin modulates the T-cell immune response and reverses starvation-induced immunosuppression', *Nature* 394 (1998): 897–901; G Fantuzzi and R Faggioni, 'Leptin in the regulation of immunity, inflammation, and hematopoiesis', *Journal of Leukocyte Biology* 68 (2000): 437–46.

223. Klok et al, 'The role of leptin and ghrelin'.

224. Klok et al, 'The role of leptin and ghrelin'.

225. M Berger et al., 'The expanded biology of serotonin', *Annual Review of Medicine* 60 (2009): 355–66; T C Birdsall, '5-Hydroxytryptophan: A clinically-effective serotonin precursor', *Alternative Medicine Review* 3, no. 4 (August 1998): 271–80.

226. D Mendelsohn et al., 'Effects of acute tryptophan depletion on memory, attention and executive functions: A systematic review', *Neuroscience and Biobehavioral Review* 33, no. 6 (June 2009): 926–52.

227. C Lassale, G D Batty, A Baghdadli, et al., 'Healthy dietary indices and risk of depressive outcomes: A systematic review and meta-analysis of observational studies', *Molecular Psychiatry* 24 (2019): 965–86; L Schwingshackl, C Schwedhelm, C Galbete, and G Hoffmann, 'Adherence to Mediterranean diet and risk of cancer: An updated systematic review and meta-analysis', *Nutrients* 9, no. 10 (2017): 1063, doi: 10.3390/nu9101063; N Veronese et al., 'Adherence to a Mediterranean diet is associated with lower incidence of frailty: A longitudinal cohort study', *Clinical Nutrition* 37, no. 5 (October 2018): 1492–97; N Veronese, et al. 'Adherence to a Mediterranean diet is associated with lower prevalence of osteoarthritis: Data from the osteoarthritis initiative', *Clinical Nutrition* 37, no. 6 (2017): 1609–14; R Widmer et al., 'The Mediterranean diet, its components, and cardiovascular disease', *American Journal of Medicine* 128, no. 3 (2015): 229–38.

228. H J Challa, M A Ameer, and K R Uppaluri, 'DASH diet to stop hypertension,' National Center for Biotechnology Information, last updated 23 May 2020, https://www.ncbi.nlm.nih.gov/books/NBK482514.

229. S Almoosawi et al., 'Chrono- nutrition: A review of current evidence from observational studies on global trends in time-of-day of energy intake and its association with obesity', *Proceedings of the Nutrition Society* 75 (2016): 487–500.

230. L C Ruddick-Collins et al., 'The big breakfast study: Chrono-nutrition influence on energy expenditure and bodyweight', *Nutrition Bulletin* 43 (2018): 174–83.

231. L Antunes, R Levandovski, G Dantas, et al., 'Obesity and shift work: Chronobiological aspects', *Nutrition Research Reviews* 23 (2010): 155–68; D M Arble, J Bass, A D Laposky, et al., 'Circadian timing of food intake contributes to weight gain', *Obesity* 17 (2009): 2100–2102; J Cleator, J Abbott, P Judd, et al., 'Night eating syndrome: Implications for severe obesity', *Nutrition and Diabetes* 2 (2012): e44; M Fong, I D Caterson, and C D Madigan, 'Are large dinners associated with excess weight, and does eating a smaller dinner achieve greater weight loss? A systematic review and meta-analysis', *British Journal of Nutrition* 118 (2017): 616–28; M Garaulet, P Gomez-Abellan, J J Alburquerque-Bejar, et al., 'Timing of food intake predicts weight loss effectiveness', *International Journal of Obesity* 37 (2013): 604–11; D Jakubowicz, M Barnea, J Wainstein, et al., 'High caloric intake at breakfast vs. dinner differentially influences weight loss of overweight and obese women', *Obesity* 21 (2013): 2504–12; D Jakubowicz, J Wainstein, Z Landau, et al., 'Influences of breakfast on clock gene expression and postprandial glycemia in healthy individuals and individuals with diabetes: A randomized clinical trial', *Diabetes Care* 40 (2017): 1573–79; Y Ma, E R Bertone, E J Stanek III, et al., 'Association between eating patterns and obesity in a free-living US adult population', *American Journal of Epidemiology* 158 (2003): 85–92; A W McHill, A J Phillips, C A Czeisler, et al., 'Later circadian timing of food intake is associated with increased body fat', *American Journal of Clinical Nutrition* 106 (2017): 1213–19; F A Scheer, M F Hilton, C S Mantzoros, et al., 'Adverse metabolic and cardiovascular consequences of circadian misalignment', *Proceedings of the National Academy of Sciences of the United States of America* 106 (2009): 4453–58; Ruddick-Collins, 'The big breakfast study'.

232. D Jakubowicz et al., 'High caloric intake at breakfast vs. dinner differentially influences weight loss of overweight and obese women', *Obesity* 21 (2013): 2504–12.

233. Ruddick-Collins, 'The big breakfast study'; C Mahoney, 'The acute effects of meals on cognitive performance', in *Nutritional Neuroscience*, ed. H R Lieberman, R B Kanarek, and C Prasad (Boca Raton, FL: Taylor & Francis Group, 2005) 73–91; A Jacques et al., 'The impact of sugar consumption on stress driven, emotional and addictive behaviours', *Neuroscience and Biobehavioural Reviews* 103 (2019): 178–99.

234. Ruddick-Collins et al., 'The big breakfast study'; Mahoney, 'Acute effects of meals on cognitive performance'; Y Akitsuki et al., 'Nutritional quality of breakfast affects cognitive function: An fMRI study', *Neuroscience and Medicine* 2 (2011): 192–97.

235. E Sutton et al., 'Early time-restricted feeding improves insulin sensitivity, blood pressure, and oxidative stress even without weight loss in men with prediabetes', *Cell Metabolism* 27 (2018): 1212–21; P Regmi and L K Heilbronn, 'Time-restricted eating: Benefits, mechanisms, and challenges in translation', *Science* 23, no. 6 (2020): 101161, doi: 10.1016/j.isci.2020.101161.

236. Sutton et al., 'Early time-restricted feeding'.

237. J Lykkesfeldt, A J Michels, and B Frei, 'Vitamin C', *Advances in Nutrition* 5, no. 1 (2014): 16–18.

238. H Hemilä and E Chalker, 'Vitamin C for preventing and treating the common cold', *Cochrane Database of Systematic Reviews* 1 (31 January 2013): CD000980, doi: 10.1002/14651858.CD000980.pub4.

239. J Suez et al., 'The pros, cons, and many unknowns of probiotics', *Nature Medicine* 25 (2019): 716–29; G Wieërs, L Belkhir, R Enaud, et al., 'How probiotics affect the microbiota', *Frontiers in Cellular and Infection Microbiology* 9 (15 January 2020): 454, doi: 10.3389/fcimb.2019.00454.

240. M Pulido-Moran, J Moreno-Fernandez, C Ramirez-Tortosa, M Ramirez-Tortosa, 'Curcumin and health', *Molecules* 21, no. 3 (25 February 2016): 264; V P Menon and A R Sudheer, 'Antioxidant and anti-inflammatory properties of curcumin', *Advances in Experimental Medicine and Biology* 595 (2007): 105–25.

241. R Kreider et al., 'International Society of Sports Nutrition position stand: Safety and efficacy of creatine supplementation in exercise, sport, and medicine', *Journal of the International Society of Sports Nutrition* 14 (13 June 2017): 18.

242. R Jäger et al., 'International Society of Sports Nutrition position stand: Probiotics', *Journal of the International Society of Sports Nutrition* 16, no. 1 (2019): 62.

## 16. Nutrition for Exercise and Recovery

243. C Kerksick et al., 'ISSN exercise and sports nutrition review update: Research and recommendations', *Journal of the International Society of Sports Nutrition* 15, no. 1 (1 August 2018): 38.

244. J Peake et al., 'Muscle damage and inflammation during recovery from exercise', *Journal of Applied Physiology* 122, no. 3 (1 March 2017): 559–70; D T Thomas, K A Erdman, and L M Burke, 'American College of Sports Medicine joint position statement: Nutrition and athletic performance', *Medicine and Science in Sports and Exercise* 48, no. 3 (March 2016): 543–68.

245. R Jäger et al., 'International Society of Sports Nutrition position stand: Protein and exercise', *Journal of the International Society of Sports Nutrition* 20 (2017): 20–45.

246. K Vitale, A Getzin, 'Nutrition and supplement update for the endurance athlete: Review and recommendations', *Nutrients* 11, no. 6 (7 June 2019): 1289.

247. Thomas, Erdman, and Burke, 'Nutrition and Athletic Performance'.

248. S Jenner et al., 'Dietary intakes of professional and semi-professional team sport athletes do not meet sport nutrition recommendations: A systematic literature review', *Nutrients* 11, no. 5 (2019): 1160; D Logue et al., 'Low energy availability in athletes 2020: An updated narrative review of prevalence, risk, within—day energy balance, knowledge, and impact on sports performance', *Nutrients* 12, no. 3 (2020): 835.

## 17. Sleep to Succeed

249. Centers for Disease Control and Prevention, 'Short sleep duration among US adults', last reviewed 2 May 2017, https://www.cdc.gov/sleep/data_statistics.html.

250. K Kochanek et al., 'Mortality in the United States, 2013', *NCHS Data Brief* 178 (2014): 1–8.

251. J L Broussard et al., 'Sleep restriction increases free fatty acids in healthy men', *Diabetologia* 58, no. 4 (April 2015): 791–98, doi:10.1007/s00125-015-3500-4.

252. M Hafner et al., 'Why sleep matters—The economic costs of insufficient sleep: A cross-country comparative analysis', *RAND Health Quarterly* 6, no. 4 (2017): 11.

253. M Hafner et al., 'Why sleep matters—the economic costs of insufficient sleep: A cross-country comparative analysis', *RAND Health Quarterly* 6, no. 4 (2017):11.

254. S Chokroverty, ed., *Sleep Disorders Medicine*, 4th ed. (New York: Springer, 2017).

255. C B Saper et al., 'Hypothalamic regulation of sleep and circadian rhythms', *Nature* 437 (2005): 1257–63.

256. S Chokroverty (ed.), *Sleep Disorders Medicine: Basic Science, Technical Considerations and Clinical Aspects*, 4th ed. (New York: Springer, 2017), 21.

257. M St-Onge et al., 'Fiber and saturated fat are associated with sleep arousals and slow wave sleep', *Journal of Clinical Sleep Medicine* 12 (2016): 19–24; M Walker, *Why We Sleep: The New Science of Sleep and Dreams* (London: Penguin, 2017).

258. M Stein et al., 'Disturbed sleep and its relationship to alcohol use', *Substance Abuse* 26 (2005): 1–13.

259. H Landolt et al., 'Late afternoon ethanol intake affects nocturnal sleep and sleep EEG in middle-aged men', *Journal of Clinical Psychopharmacology* 16 (1996): 428–36.

260. M W Chee and Y M Chuah, 'Functional neuroimaging and behavioural correlates of capacity decline in visual short-term memory after sleep deprivation', *Proceedings of the National Academy of Science* 104 (2007): 9487–92.5; P Alhola, P Polo-Kantola, 'Sleep deprivation: Impact on cognitive performance', *Neuropsychiatric Disease and Treatment* 3, no. 5 (2007): 553–67; J A Horne, *Why We Sleep: The Functions of Sleep in Humans and Other Mammals* (Oxford: Oxford University Press, 1988), 13–75; J A Horne, 'Sleep loss and "divergent" thinking ability', *Sleep* 11, no. 6 (1988): 528–36; J A Horne, 'Human sleep, sleep loss and behavior: Implications for the prefrontal cortex and psychiatric disorder', *British Journal of Psychiatry* 1632 (1993): 413–19.

261. H P A Van Dongen et al., 'The cumulative cost of additional wakefulness', *Sleep* 26, no. 2 (2003): 117–26.

262. G P Krueger, 'Fatigue, drowsy decision-making and medical error: Issues of quality health care', *Journal of the Washington Academy of Sciences* 92, no. 2 (2006): 41–60; N J Taffinder et al., 'Effect of sleep deprivation on surgeons' dexterity in a laparoscopic simulator', Lancet 352 (1998): 1191; C H M Jacques et al., 'The effects of sleep loss on cognitive performance of resident physicians', *Journal of Family Practice* 30, no. 2 (1990): 223–29.

263. D Dawson and K Reid, 'Fatigue, alcohol and performance impairment', *Nature* 388 (1997): 235.

264. M P Walker, et al., 'Practice with sleep makes perfect: Sleep-dependent motor skill learning', *Neuron* 35, no. 1 (2002): 205–11.

265. M Milewski et al., 'Chronic lack of sleep is associated with increased sports injuries in adolescent athletes', *Journal of Pediatric Orthopaedics* 34, no. 2 (March 2014): 129–33.

266. Milewski et al., 'Chronic lack of sleep is associated with increased sports injuries in adolescent athletes'.

267. L E Juliff et al., 'Longer sleep durations are positively associated with finishing place during a national multi-day netball competition', *Journal of Strength and Conditioning Research* 32, no. 1 (January 2018):189–94.

268. J Waterhouse et al., 'The role of a short post-lunch nap in improving cognitive, motor, and sprint performance in participants with partial sleep deprivation', Journal of Sports Science 25 (2007): 1557–66; S O'Donnell et al., 'The influence of match-day napping in elite female netball athletes', *International Journal of Sports Physiology and Performance* 13 (2018): 1143–48.

269. M R Rosekind et al., 'Alertness management: Strategic naps in operational settings', *Journal of Sleep Research* 4, no. S2 (December 1995): 62–66.

270. J Waterhouse et al., 'The role of a short post-lunch nap in improving cognitive, motor, and sprint performance in participants with partial sleep deprivation', *Journal of Sports Science* 25, no. 14 (2007):1557–66.

271. J S Ruggiero and N S Redeker, 'Effects of napping on sleepiness and sleep-related performance deficits in night-shift workers: A systematic review', *Biological Research for Nursing* 16 (2014): 134–42.

272. D C Clay, A S Bro, and N J Clay, 'How does travel affect NCAA basketball outcomes?' Winthrop Intelligence (24 February 2014), https://www.canr.msu.edu/csus/uploads/458/49149/How_Does_Travel_Affect_NCAA_Basketball_Outcomes__-_Winthrop_Intelligence.pdf.

273. S D Youngstedt, J A Elliott, and D F Kripke, 'Human circadian phase–response curves for exercise', *Journal of Physiology* 597 (2019): 2253–68.

274. C R Markus et al., 'Evening intake of alpha-lactalbumin increases plasma tryptophan availability and improves morning alertness and brain measures of attention', *American Journal of Clinical Nutrition* 81 (2005): 1026–33.

275. A Afaghi, H O'Connor, and C Moi Chow, 'High-glycemic-index carbohydrate meals shorten sleep onset', *American Journal of Clinical Nutrition* 85 (2007): 426–30.

276. C M Morin and R Benca, 'Chronic insomnia', *Lancet* 379 (2112): 1129–41.

## 18. Technologies in Human Performance

277. W J Gordon, A Landman, H Zhang, et al., 'Beyond validation: Getting health apps into clinical practice', *npj Digital Medicine 3*, no. 14 (2020).

278. K M Hamilton, '3 reasons for "genius bars" in health care', MedStar Health, 11 November 2016, https://www.medstarhealth.org/digitalblog/2016/11/11/3-reasons-for-genius-bars-in-health-care.

# Acknowledgements

Firstly, my thanks to the countless patients over the years, young and old, who have inspired me.

Secondly, my huge thanks and respect to Lois Stück, my wonderful copyeditor. A true professional, who has shown great patience and expertise throughout her involvement in the project.

All figures were created using biorender.com.

Cover design: VeryMuchSo.agency

My sincere thanks to Geoff Borin for his excellent assistance with book design.

Made in the USA
Monee, IL
03 November 2026

67374672R00148